Crohn's & Colitis

SECOND EDITION

SECOND EDITION

Crohn's & Colitis

Understanding & Managing IBD

Dr. A. Hillary Steinhart

MD, MSc, FRCP(C)
Division Head, Gastroenterology
Mount Sinai Hospital

Robert
ROSE

Crohn's & Colitis, Second Edition
Text copyright © 2006, 2012 A. Hillary Steinhart
Illustrations copyright © 2012 Robert Rose, Inc.
Cover and text design copyright © 2012 Robert Rose Inc.

The author would like to thank the following for sharing her knowledge and expertise during the writing of this book: Dr. Anne Griffiths, Hospital for Sick Children, Toronto, Ontario.

For complete cataloguing information, see page 228.

Disclaimer

This book is a general guide only and should never be a substitute for the skill, knowledge, and experience of a qualified medical professional dealing with the facts, circumstances, and symptoms of a particular case.

The nutritional, medical, and health information presented in this book is based on the research, training, and professional experience of the author, and is true and complete to the best of his knowledge. However, this book is intended only as an informative guide for those wishing to know more about health, nutrition, and medicine; it is not intended to replace or countermand the advice given by the reader's personal physician. Because each person and situation is unique, the author and the publisher urge the reader to check with a qualified health-care professional before using any procedure where there is a question as to its appropriateness. A physician should be consulted before beginning any exercise program. The author and the publisher are not responsible for any adverse effects or consequences resulting from the use of the information in this book. It is the responsibility of the reader to consult a physician or other qualified health-care professional regarding his or her personal care.

Design and Production: Kevin Cockburn/PageWave Graphics Inc.
Editor: Bob Hilderley, Senior Editor, Health
Proofreader: Sheila Wawanash
Indexer: Gillian Watts
Illustrations: Kveta/Three in a Box
Cover image: © iStockphoto.com/Juan Facundo Mora Soria

We acknowledge the financial support of the Government of Canada through the Book Publishing Industry Development Program (BPIDP) for our publishing activities.

Published by Robert Rose Inc.
120 Eglinton Avenue East, Suite 800, Toronto, Ontario, Canada M4P 1E2
Tel: (416) 322-6552 Fax: (416) 322-6936
www.robertrose.ca

Printed and bound in Canada

1 2 3 4 5 6 7 8 9 TGILBF 20 19 18 17 16 15 14 13 12

Contents

PART 2 • Managing Inflammatory Bowel Disease

Preface

Living with inflammatory bowel disease (IBD) can be a challenge, not only for those of you who have Crohn's disease or ulcerative colitis, but also for those of you who have a family member or close friend afflicted with one of these disorders. Meeting this challenge requires the help of knowledgeable health-care professionals. Knowing yourself what impact Crohn's disease and ulcerative colitis may have on your life and what management strategies are available is also very important. The well-informed patient may have the best chance for recovery.

However, the amount of information you can find when trying to learn about inflammatory bowel disease can be overwhelming. There are so many possible sources of information — doctors, nurses, books, pamphlets, websites, patient associations, Internet chat rooms, friends, and relatives. Often this information is confusing and contradictory. The quality of the information varies greatly from source to source. This information overload can leave you confused and frustrated, thus making it even more difficult to deal with these chronic diseases.

We have written this book in order to provide patients, families, friends, and health-care professionals with a clear, current, and concise account of the possible underlying causes, clinical features, and effective treatments of Crohn's disease and ulcerative colitis. Rather than simply presenting a list of facts about the disorders, we have given them an applied clinical context based upon our years of experience with many hundreds of patients who have been evaluated, followed, and treated at the Mount Sinai Hospital IBD Centre. We have also tried to make this information directly relevant to IBD sufferers and their families by recounting case histories and answering the questions patients frequently ask. We hope to provide another means for dealing with these diseases, which we are only now really beginning to understand.

> We have written this book in order to provide patients, families, friends, and health-care professionals with a clear, current, and concise account of the possible underlying causes, clinical features, and effective treatments of Crohn's disease and ulcerative colitis.

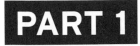

PART 1

UNDERSTANDING CROHN'S DISEASE

AND

ULCERATIVE COLITIS

CHAPTER 1

What Is This Disease?

CASE STUDY Kelly

Kelly, a 22-year-old university student, developed symptoms of abdominal cramping, urgency to move her bowels, diarrhea, and blood in the stool. The symptoms came on gradually and were at first intermittent. They began during the month before her first-term exams, and, although they seemed to improve after she finished the exams, the symptoms continued into the second term. She went to the university health clinic, where she was examined and referred to a specialist. The specialist carried out some tests and told Kelly that she had inflammatory bowel disease, specifically, ulcerative colitis.

Kelly was really upset — ulcerative colitis sounded like a serious disease. Besides, the doctor told her there is no cure, other than surgery. It wasn't fair. "I'm young," she protested, "and no one in my family has had this disease. I've always been very health conscious… I eat a healthy diet, including milk and dairy products. I'm physically active and I don't smoke." She couldn't stop asking questions in her effort to understand why. "What is inflammatory bowel disease? Is colitis an infection? Can I take antibiotics to cure it? Did the stress of my exams cause it? What if I eat a different diet? Could the ibuprofen I take for headaches have an impact?"

Her doctor calmed her down and began answering Kelly's questions…

(continued on page 56)

Inflammation Location

In Crohn's disease, inflammation occurs most often in the lower part of the small intestine, called the ileum, and the large intestine, also known as the colon. Crohn's disease can also affect the esophagus, stomach, and upper parts of the small intestine (duodenum and jejunum).

What Is Inflammatory Bowel Disease?

Inflammatory bowel disease is not a single disease or medical condition. The term describes, in a general way, any condition or disease that results in inflammation of the gastrointestinal tract. Strictly speaking, this definition would include infections of the intestine, for example, infection caused by salmonella bacteria. However, the term "inflammatory bowel disease" (IBD) is usually reserved for two similar disorders, Crohn's disease and ulcerative colitis. Specific causes for these disorders are not yet entirely known.

Crohn's Disease

Crohn's disease probably dates back to the early 19th century, based upon descriptions of cases of similar ailments in the medical literature of that era. In 1932, Drs. Crohn, Ginzburg, and Oppenheimer at the Mount Sinai Hospital in New York first described the condition as a specific disease entity. The form of the disease they originally described focused on inflammation of the ileum, the last part of the small intestine. They called the condition "regional ileitis," with "ileitis" indicating inflammation of the ileum. Several years after Dr. Crohn and colleagues described the condition, it was given the name "Crohn's disease." In the early 1950s, it was recognized that Crohn's disease did not necessarily affect just the ileum, but that other parts of the gastrointestinal tract, such as the colon or large intestine, could be affected.

Ulcerative Colitis

Like Crohn's disease, ulcerative colitis had probably been with us for some time before it was fully described in the late 19th century. Ulcerative colitis is sometimes referred to as "ulcerative proctitis," "ulcerative proctosigmoiditis," or "ulcerative pancolitis." These names relate primarily to the extent of the inflammation of the colon rather than to any fundamental differences in the presumed causes of ulcerative colitis. In the first half of the 20th century, the treatment of ulcerative colitis was surgical, and many patients ended up dying of complications of the disease or the surgery. Since the 1940s, there has been a consistent improvement in the surgical and medical management of ulcerative colitis, and death due to complications of the disease or its treatment is now exceedingly rare.

| **Limited Inflammation** |
| In ulcerative colitis, the inflammation is limited to the large intestine, which includes the rectum. The rest of the gastrointestinal tract is not involved. |

Irritable Bowel Syndrome

Inflammatory bowel disease (IBD) and irritable bowel syndrome (IBS) are often confused since their names are so alike. IBS is a poorly understood condition of the gastrointestinal tract. Although IBS is characterized by chronic abdominal discomfort or pain and an alteration in the normal bowel habit, it is quite a different condition from Crohn's disease and ulcerative colitis (IBD).

In IBS, it is thought that the problems arise from a change in the way the bowel functions or the way in which the brain senses the bowel functioning. In IBS, there has been no clear or consistent evidence that inflammation plays a role in causing the symptoms in humans. This is different from IBD, where inflammation is the main defining characteristic of the disease, and where treatment against inflammation will help the disease and its symptoms. In IBS, treatment is usually aimed at modifying the motility of the gastrointestinal tract or the transmission of the pain impulses from the intestine to the brain.

Glossary of Inflammatory Bowel Disease

Gastroenterologists use several technical terms to describe IBD. You can start to use the language of this disease in discussions with your health-care providers. These terms are defined more thoroughly in their context later in the book.

Abscess: a localized collection of dead and infected tissue (pus), which typically becomes liquid. The consequences may be serious if it is not quickly and properly managed; management involves draining the infected material and treating with antibiotics.

Absorption: the digestive process of extracting nutrients from food and transferring these nutrients into the circulatory system; for example, the absorption of foods containing vitamin B_{12} occurs in the ileum (the last section of the small intestine), which is often problematic in IBD.

Anal sphincter: a muscular valve at the bottom of the rectum, which normally prevents stool from coming out when it is not supposed to. Damage to the sphincter or the nerves supplying the sphincter can lead to fecal incontinence.

Colon (large intestine): the lower part of the gastrointestinal tract, which is primarily responsible for reabsorbing fluid and electrolytes (salts) from the stool.

Colonoscopy: a diagnostic procedure for IBD, which involves inserting a scope through the anus and rectum to the colon, where a tissue biopsy may be taken for testing.

Distension: a significant increase in the size of the abdomen may be due to gas, stool or fluid.

Duodenum: the first part of the small intestine, which receives ingested food after it has left the stomach. Although the duodenum is relatively short (about 1 foot/30 cm in length), it has an important role in the absorption of some nutrients, particularly iron; it is also the location where digestive enzymes from the pancreas and bile salts from the liver are first mixed together with food in order to help the digestion process.

Enzyme: a protein that helps the rate of a chemical reaction, usually related to an important metabolic function of the body.

Fecal incontinence: loss of the ability to hold stool (fecal waste). This may happen from time to time or, in some cases, on a regular basis.

Fistula: an abnormal communication or channel from the intestine to other organs or to the abdominal wall or skin.

Gastroenterology: a medical specialty involved in the study of the digestive system, digestive disease, and digestive health.

Gastrointestinal (GI) tract: extends from the mouth to the anus.

Granuloma: a distinctive collection of inflammatory or immune cells that occur in tissues affected by certain conditions, including Crohn's disease.

Ileum: the last part of the small intestine; makes up about one-third of the entire length of the small intestine. Vitamin B_{12} is absorbed here.

Inflammatory bowel disease (IBD): any condition or disease that results in inflammation of the gastrointestinal tract, most commonly in the small and large intestine and the rectum.

Irritable bowel syndrome (IBS): a functional GI syndrome characterized by inflammation, infection, and bacterial changes in the gut but not restricted to any one organ.

Jejunum: the second part of the small intestine, which makes up about two-thirds of the entire length of the small intestine and is responsible for the absorption of most of the nutrients from food.

Lymphocyte: a type of white blood cell that is important in immune protection against a number of different possible bacteria and viruses that can cause infection.

Motility: the movement of food through the GI tract.

Mucosa: the inner lining of the gastrointestinal tract. The integrity of the mucosa is important for carrying out many of the roles of the gastrointestinal tract, particularly digestion of food and absorption of nutrients.

Pancolitis: inflammation that involves the entire colon.

Perforation: a hole in the wall of the intestine, which allows intestinal contents, often with numerous bacteria, into the abdominal cavity, where serious infection may result.

Peristalsis: the involuntary contractions that move food through the GI tract.

Proctitis: a form of colitis that affects only the rectum.

Proteins: compounds made up of long-chain amino acids. Proteins are responsible for many critical functions, including maintenance of bodily structure and metabolic functions.

Rectum: the very last part of the colon (large intestine), where stool is held before it is expelled. Inflammation of the rectum can result in difficulty holding stool for extended periods of time.

Serosa: the outer lining (membrane) that covers the intestine.

Stricture: a narrowing of the central channel in a segment of the intestine, which can lead to obstruction or blockage.

Ulcer: an area in the gastrointestinal tract where there is a loss of the normal internal lining (mucosa). Ulcers can result in complications, such as bleeding or abscesses.

Villi: finger-like projections of the inner lining of the small intestine (mucosa), which they have the effect of increasing the amount of mucosal surface available for absorption of nutrients.

Smoking Paradox

Smoking seems to increase the risk of Crohn's disease, and in those already affected, smoking may make the disease more aggressive or severe. In contrast, smoking seems to protect against ulcerative colitis. Patients with ulcerative colitis are more likely to be non-smokers or former smokers than a similar group of people selected from the general population. In former smokers, the period soon after smoking cessation seems to be a time of particularly increased risk of developing ulcerative colitis. This observation has led some researchers to use nicotine, in the form of skin patches, as a treatment for ulcerative colitis. Despite the strong association between cigarette smoking and protection against ulcerative colitis, this approach to treatment has not been consistently effective.

Who Gets Inflammatory Bowel Disease?

The onset of inflammatory bowel disease may be influenced by age, gender, and geography.

Age Factors

Crohn's disease and ulcerative colitis most commonly begin in young people. Although it is unusual to see this disorder in children below the age of 5, there is an increase in the occurrence of IBD up until the age of 20, with maximum incidence in the age group between 20 and 40. It is less common, but certainly not unheard of, for older individuals in their 50s and 60s to first experience IBD. First onset of disease is quite rare in the elderly. When symptoms first occur in someone from that age group, the attending doctor will usually consider other conditions or illnesses as more likely than IBD.

Gender

Inflammatory bowel disease appears to occur in males and females at roughly the same rate, although some studies have suggested that there may be slightly higher incidence in females. These differences may vary depending on the age of the first onset of IBD, but even if such differences exist, they are likely to be minor and of no major significance.

Population Studies

Although they are generally thought to be diseases that are found more frequently in developed countries, Crohn's disease and ulcerative colitis have been observed in every ethnic group that has been specifically studied. There do appear to be some interesting differences between countries, as well as between ethnic groups within a given country.

These diseases are much less common in Asia, but this may be changing. In Japan, for example, Crohn's disease was almost unheard of 50 years ago, but there appears to have been a steady increase in the incidence since then. The incidence in the Jewish population is among the highest of any ethnic or racial group. However, within the Jewish population there appears to be a difference in incidence depending upon the country of origin. In one study, the incidence of IBD was higher in Jews of Ashkenazi (European) descent than in Jewish populations of Sephardic (Northern African and Middle Eastern) descent.

The varying risks of IBD in different countries are not entirely due to purely inherited or genetic reasons. The increasing incidence of Crohn's disease observed in Japan suggests that environmental factors have an important effect on the risk of developing IBD. In addition, studies of South Asian immigrants to North America have shown that the individuals who immigrate keep the lower risk of IBD that is seen in their country of origin, whereas their children, who are generally born and raised in North America, have a higher risk of developing IBD in their lifetime. These variations in the incidence of IBD provide clues as to the possible contributing factors or causes and have led to a number of interesting theories and questions that are undergoing further testing.

North-South Gradient

The incidence of IBD has generally been highest in North America and Northern European countries and lower in the countries at more southerly latitudes. This has been described as a "north-south gradient."

Where in the Body Does IBD Occur?

Inflammatory bowel disease occurs in specific sections of the gastrointestinal tract, or gut. Before considering what has gone wrong in Crohn's disease and ulcerative colitis, we need to understand how a healthy gut works. The normal functioning of the intestinal immune system may go awry in inflammatory bowel disease.

Functions of the Gastrointestinal Tract

The gastrointestinal tract is a tubular structure that extends from the mouth all the way down to the anus. The gut has two vital functions — nutrient absorption and immune protection.

Critical for Life

The gastrointestinal tract serves several critical functions that help to keep us alive. It allows nutrients, water, minerals, and vitamins to enter our body while keeping out harmful substances.

Principal Parts of the Gastrointestinal Tract

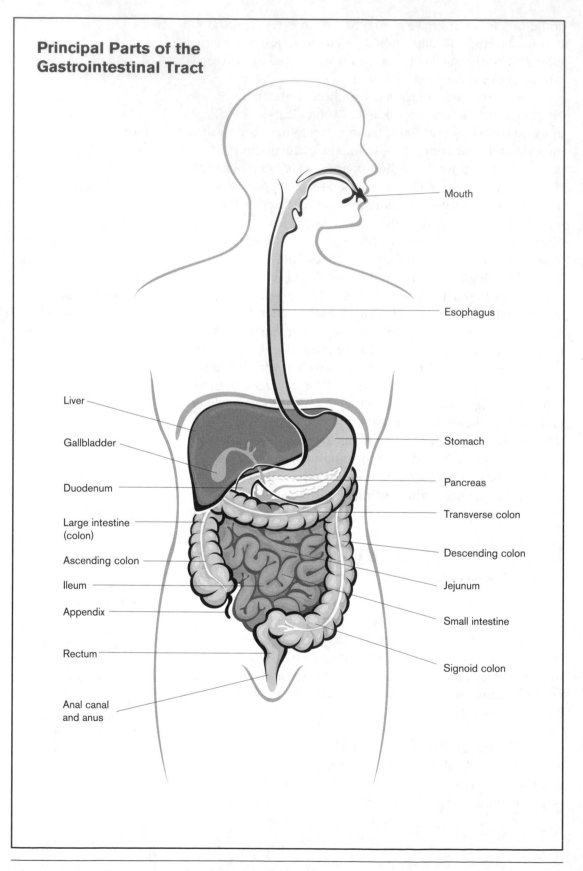

Mouth

Esophagus

Liver

Gallbladder

Stomach

Duodenum

Pancreas

Large intestine (colon)

Transverse colon

Ascending colon

Descending colon

Ileum

Jejunum

Appendix

Small intestine

Rectum

Signoid colon

Anal canal and anus

Nutrient Absorption

The primary job of the gut is to take in and absorb nutrients. These nutrients provide the building blocks and fuel needed to maintain all other bodily functions. The gut absorbs water, minerals, and vitamins from the food and drinks that are ingested.

Immune Protection

At the same time that it allows or promotes absorption of nutrients, the gastrointestinal tract must keep numerous potentially harmful items out of the body. These include microscopic organisms, such as bacteria, viruses, and parasites, as well as certain dangerous proteins that may cause disease if absorbed into the body from the gut. The gastrointestinal tract is, therefore, an important part of the body's immune system.

Principal Parts of the Gastrointestinal Tract

The gastrointestinal tract has seven major components: mouth, esophagus, stomach, small intestine, large intestine, and anus. The esophagus, stomach, small intestine, mucosa, large intestine, and anus may all be affected by inflammatory bowel disease.

Mouth

The mouth and the structures within it (lips, teeth, tongue and palate) are involved in the ingestion of food. The teeth allow the grinding of food into small particles that are more easily broken down and digested by the enzymes present further down in the intestine. The lips, tongue, and palate assist with the chewing and swallowing of food.

Esophagus

The esophagus (or gullet) is a tube that transports food, once it is swallowed, from the mouth to the stomach. A valve at the bottom of the esophagus prevents food and stomach acid from coming back up into the esophagus and into the mouth, where it can cause heartburn, which can result in damage to the inner lining of the esophagus. When you vomit, this valve opens up to allow acid and food to come out, and when you burp, it opens to allow gas to come out.

Stomach

This sac-like structure lies in the upper part of the abdomen. It receives and holds food that has recently been eaten and slowly pushes it down into the small intestine, where most of the absorption of nutrients occurs. There is a valve at the lower end of the stomach that helps to regulate how quickly the food leaves the stomach to enter the small intestine. The stomach

---

IBD Ulcers

An area that has lost its mucosal lining is called an ulcer. When people talk about ulcers, they are usually referring to duodenal or gastric (stomach) ulcers, which are typically different from the ulcers that may occur in inflammatory bowel disease. In Crohn's disease and ulcerative colitis, the ulcers usually occur in the small intestine and large intestine and much less commonly in the stomach and duodenum.

---

provides an important signal to the brain to indicate when you have eaten enough.

The stomach also secretes acid from its lining. This helps to protect against infections caused by harmful bacteria that might inadvertently be ingested during a meal. The stomach acid also helps with the initial digestion of proteins in food, secreting an enzyme, called pepsin, that helps with the breakdown of proteins.

Small Intestine

The small intestine (or small bowel) is a tubular structure approximately 12 to 15 feet (4 to 5 m) long. It is divided into three segments: from top to bottom, these are the duodenum, the jejunum, and the ileum. In the small intestine, most of the nutrients in food are absorbed into the body.

Mucosa

The absorption of nutrients is dependent upon the presence of a highly specialized inner lining (or mucosa). The mucosa lining is made up of cells whose main reason for being is to absorb nutrients from the inside (or lumen) of the intestine and pass them through into the body, where they are available as building blocks or fuel for other body functions. The surface of the mucosa is folded into many tiny finger-like projections, called villi, which effectively increase the surface area and, therefore, the number of cells available for absorption of nutrients.

The surface of these cells contains enzymes that help break down food into smaller components so as to be absorbed more easily. When the intestine is inflamed, as is the case in inflammatory bowel disease, the villi may be reduced in number or size — or may be wiped out altogether so that the inner lining of the intestine appears flat. This loss of normal villi results in reduced ability to absorb nutrients. When the inflammation is severe, the mucosa lining may be completely gone, leaving the underlying tissue exposed to the inside of the intestine.

Large Intestine

The large intestine, also known as the colon, is approximately 3 to 4 feet (1 to 1.2 m) in length. Although shorter than the small intestine, it is called the large intestine because its width or diameter is greater than that of the small intestine. It is divided into several sections: cecum, ascending colon, transverse colon, descending colon, sigmoid colon, and rectum.

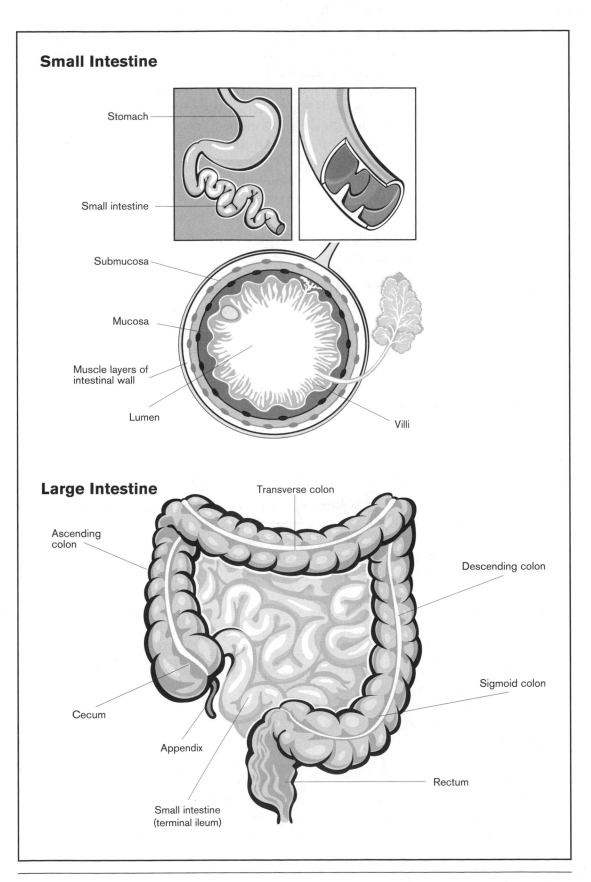

Small Intestine

Stomach

Small intestine

Submucosa

Mucosa

Muscle layers of intestinal wall

Lumen

Villi

Large Intestine

Transverse colon

Ascending colon

Descending colon

Cecum

Sigmoid colon

Appendix

Rectum

Small intestine (terminal ileum)

Rectum

The last part of the large intestine is called the rectum. The wall of the rectum can stretch, up to a certain point, to allow stool to be kept inside until there is an appropriate time to evacuate. When the rectum is inflamed or somehow diseased in other ways, that ability to hold stool is reduced, and you may feel the need to go to the bathroom very frequently and urgently. In some instances, this can result in accidents with associated loss of control of bowel function, otherwise known as fecal incontinence. This need for frequent bathroom visits and the urgency that may go along with it can be one of the most troubling symptoms of inflammatory bowel disease.

Related Parts of the Gastrointestinal Tract

There are other parts of the gastrointestinal tract involved to a greater or lesser extent in digestion and nutrient absorption. These organs, which are typically connected to the tubular part of the gastrointestinal tract by small channels (or ducts), include the liver, gallbladder, and pancreas. The gallbladder and pancreas are usually not affected by inflammatory bowel disease. However, the liver may be affected in a small proportion of patients. Rarely, this can lead to liver damage.

Liver

The liver has many functions, but the one that is most involved in digestion is bile production. Bile is similar to a detergent, in that it allows fat to be broken down and made into a form that can be dissolved or mixed with water. Normally, fat remains separate from water, like the fat floating on the top of chicken soup. This ability of bile to break up fat into small particles and disperse those particles in the watery contents of the small intestine is crucial to fat digestion and absorption.

Gallbladder

Bile that is produced by the liver is usually stored in the gallbladder, a small sac next to the liver, until it is needed after a meal. When the production of bile is not adequate or if bile is blocked from reaching the intestine, absorption of fat from the diet is reduced. As a result, fat may end up coming out in the stool. This appears as droplets of fat or oil in the stool.

Pancreas

The pancreas is a gland producing a number of digestive enzymes that enter the upper part of the small intestine. The pancreas lies very close to the duodenum and has a small duct running through it that carries the enzymes from the pancreas into the duodenum. These enzymes help break down protein, starch, and fat in the diet into components that can be easily absorbed by the intestine.

Anus

The anus (or anal canal) is the passageway that stool follows when it leaves the body. The primary role of the anus is to keep the stool that is present in the rectum from coming out when you don't want it to come out. In other words, it helps to prevent fecal incontinence. Within the anal canal, there are two main muscular anal sphincters (or valves) that help to prevent the stool from coming out involuntarily.

One of the sphincters, called the external anal sphincter, is under your conscious control. In other words, you can control or tighten this particular sphincter when trying to hold in stool or gas. The other sphincter, the internal anal sphincter, is not under voluntary control, but works reflexively at a subconscious level. Maintaining continence and ensuring the smooth and complete emptying of the rectum requires the coordination of the two anal sphincters. If either of these two sphincters is damaged or diseased, it can result in fecal incontinence.

What Goes Wrong in the Gut with IBD?

Crohn's disease and ulcerative colitis involve inflammation of the gut. A healthy person normally has a certain degree of inflammation in the gastrointestinal tract, but in those with IBD, the inflammation is extensive and excessive.

Normal Intestinal Inflammation

In the gut, the degree of inflammation that is normally present in healthy people is usually not enough to cause loss of function or to be seen by the naked eye, but when viewed under the magnification provided by a microscope, you can always see some white blood cells, called lymphocytes, present within the lining and just beneath the lining of the intestine.

These defensive cells are part of the intestine's immune system that help to protect you from potentially harmful bacteria, viruses, parasites, and proteins that aren't normally present in the body. The amount of inflammation is closely regulated so that there is just enough immune response so as to protect against these dangers, but not so much that it will cause problems.

Too much of a good thing may be bad, and the amount of inflammation in the intestinal lining is no exception. If there is too much inflammation or if it is not properly controlled, inflammation can cause swelling and damage to the tissues of the gastrointestinal tract. This damage can lead to problems with the normal functioning of the gastrointestinal tract, including absorption of nutrients and fluids and retaining and expelling stool at appropriate times.

When the damage is particularly severe, the internal lining of the gastrointestinal tract can slough off, leading to a variety of symptoms, such as abdominal pain, diarrhea, blood in the stool, weight loss, and failure of children to grow properly.

Ulcerative Colitis Signs

Inflammation in ulcerative colitis is limited to the colon, but the extent of the inflammation within the colon varies from person to person and may vary within an individual over the course of the illness.

Any portion of the colon may be inflamed in ulcerative colitis, leaving the remainder completely unaffected. However, the rectum is always inflamed or diseased.

Pancolitis

In many instances, the entire colon is inflamed. This is referred to as pancolitis. When the inflammation extends upwards, it does so in a continuous fashion. In other words, there are no areas of inflammation separated from one another by normal areas of colon.

Proctitis

In some people with ulcerative colitis, only the rectum is inflamed. This particular form of the disease is often referred to as proctitis or ulcerative proctitis. Some differences have been observed between proctitis and the more extensive forms of the disease, such as pancolitis. Ulcerative proctitis is unusual in children and tends to be seen more often when the disease occurs for the first time in middle-aged or elderly individuals.

Crohn's Disease Signs

In Crohn's disease, the inflammation can occur in any part of the gastrointestinal tract. Although it appears most often in the ileum and colon, Crohn's disease can affect the esophagus, stomach, duodenum, and jejunum.

Skip Lesions

The areas of the gut affected by Crohn's disease may not be adjacent to one another. These are called skip lesions. For example, someone with Crohn's disease may have an area of inflammation in the middle part of the small intestine (jejunum) and another area of inflammation in the large intestine, with normal intestine in between the two areas of inflammation.

Limited Extent

Because the extent of inflammation in ulcerative proctitis is so limited — involving at most just the last 6 inches (15 cm) of the large intestine — patients suffering from that form of the disease are usually not as sick as patients with more extensive forms of ulcerative colitis.

Intestinal Penetration

In ulcerative colitis, the inflammation tends to be limited to the innermost lining of the gut, but in Crohn's disease, the inflammation has a tendency to penetrate from the innermost lining, where inflammation and ulcers first occur, right through the deeper layers of the bowel to the outer surface (serosa). This results in a defect or hole in the bowel wall, which can lead to localized infections in the abdominal cavity (abscesses) or communications (fistulas) from the bowel into other organs or into the abdominal wall or skin. The inflammation in Crohn's disease may also form into tiny localized collections of inflammatory cells, called granulomas, which can be seen only under the magnification provided by a microscope. These granulomas are virtually diagnostic of Crohn's disease.

Indeterminate Colitis Signs

In a small proportion of individuals with inflammatory bowel disease involving the colon, it is not possible, based upon the disease features, to differentiate between ulcerative colitis and Crohn's disease. In these instances, the condition is designated as indeterminate colitis or inflammatory bowel disease of undetermined type (IBDU). In some cases of indeterminate colitis, the pattern of disease will change over time, and it will become apparent that the patient, in fact, has ulcerative colitis or Crohn's disease. However, some patients will continue to have features of both ulcerative colitis and Crohn's disease, and distinguishing between the two will not be possible.

To some extent, the differentiation is not critical because many of the medical treatments for the two conditions are the same. Differentiation becomes much more important if surgery is contemplated as a means of treatment because the surgical approaches in ulcerative colitis and Crohn's disease can be quite different.

What Are the Possible Complications of IBD?

There are several serious complications that can occur as a result of having inflammatory bowel disease. This is where the danger lies. Some complications are common to Crohn's disease and ulcerative colitis, whereas others are unique to one form of IBD or the other. Generally, the complications can be divided into those that occur directly from the inflammation or ulceration that occurs in the intestine and those that occur in areas of the body that are not directly connected to the intestine or directly related to the intestinal inflammation.

Site Variation

The wide variation in the sites of the gut that are affected by Crohn's disease can lead to important differences in the ways individual patients experience the disease and the ways in which they come to medical attention. This variation in sites also affects approaches to management of the disease.

Complications Specific to Crohn's Disease

- Strictures
- Abscesses
- Fistulas

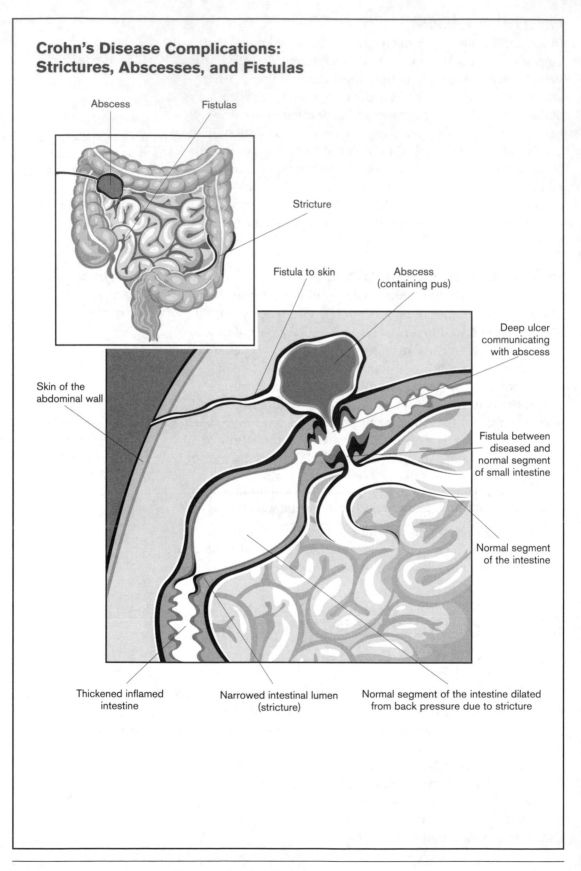

Crohn's Disease Complications: Strictures, Abscesses, and Fistulas

Abscess

Fistulas

Stricture

Fistula to skin

Abscess (containing pus)

Deep ulcer communicating with abscess

Skin of the abdominal wall

Fistula between diseased and normal segment of small intestine

Normal segment of the intestine

Thickened inflamed intestine

Narrowed intestinal lumen (stricture)

Normal segment of the intestine dilated from back pressure due to stricture

Q **What are strictures?**

A Strictures are segments of the intestine in which the normally large internal opening becomes narrowed. This can be due to the swelling that occurs in the tissues of the intestinal wall as a result of active inflammation, similar to the swelling you get when you experience an injury, such as a broken bone. More often, the stricture is due to scarring of the intestinal tissues following repeated or ongoing episodes of inflammation and healing.

Inflammation and Ulceration Complications

Inflammation and ulcerations can lead to strictures, fistulas, and abscesses in the gut. If these complications are not properly managed, they can, in turn, lead to further tissue damage and uncontrolled infection. Death can occur if this happens. While these complications are often seen in Crohn's disease, they are very rare in ulcerative colitis.

Strictures

Strictures are not necessarily a problem until they cause a bowel obstruction, commonly referred to as a blockage. Food or other material becomes caught in the narrowed stricture, preventing anything else from passing through. This produces back pressure in the intestine "upstream" from the stricture, causing sharp, often crampy pain, a distended abdomen, and nausea and vomiting. Sometimes there may be warning signs that a stricture may be worsening or leading to an obstruction. These signs include frequent or recurrent pain in the center of the abdomen after eating, along with a feeling of distension or bloating of the abdomen.

Foods to Avoid When You Have an Intestinal Stricture

- Popcorn
- Nuts
- Seeds
- Corn
- Raw vegetables
- Skins on fruits

Bowel Obstruction

Not everyone with a stricture develops intestinal obstruction. If you experience a bowel obstruction that is not severe and know the symptoms, you can sometimes manage it on your own by avoiding solid food and drinking only fluids for several hours or even a few days. If you have a stricture, it is important that you avoid eating foods that aren't easily digested and that, as a result, may get lodged in the narrowed part of the intestine. These foods include popcorn, nuts, seeds, corn, raw vegetables (particularly stringy ones like celery), and skins on fruits.

This complication can be an emergency situation. You will usually require monitoring in a hospital setting, with intravenous fluids given to prevent dehydration and possibly

Bowel Obstruction Symptoms

- Crampy severe pain, usually in the center of the abdomen
- Distension or bloating of the abdomen
- Reduced number of bowel motions
- Not passing gas
- Nausea and vomiting

Not all symptoms are necessarily present when a bowel obstruction has occurred, particularly if it is partial or incomplete.

the insertion of a nasogastric tube (a plastic tube inserted through the nose and down the esophagus into the stomach) to take fluid and gas out of the stomach.

If the obstruction does not settle with these measures, then surgery is usually required to remove the strictured area of bowel. Fortunately, most obstructions that are due to Crohn's disease strictures settle without the immediate need for surgery, but repeated obstructions usually mean that surgery is required. In that instance, the surgery can be scheduled electively so that it is performed when you are well nourished, not sick, and not on medications that might affect healing and recovery after surgery. Medications are not very effective at relieving obstruction, particularly when the narrowing is due to scarring.

Abscesses

When a deep ulcer penetrates through all of the layers of the intestine, the contents of the intestine, primarily bacteria and fecal material, can leak out and into the abdominal cavity and tissues around the intestine. When a lot of this material leaks out suddenly, it can produce a serious, and occasionally fatal, infection called peritonitis.

In Crohn's disease, this leakage normally occurs very gradually, and the tissues around the intestine have a chance to react and to form a barrier against free leakage of the bacteria into the abdominal cavity. As a result, the bacteria accumulate in a localized area that is effectively walled off. The bacteria grow in the center of this walled-off region, causing a localized infection known as an abscess. An abscess typically contains pus in its center.

Fistulas

Fistulas are abnormal channels or tracts joining one part of the intestine to another part of the intestine or to another organ. When an area of the intestine becomes inflamed and ulcerated, the ulcer can penetrate through the full thickness of the intestine wall into an adjacent tissue. This is promoted by the fact that inflamed intestine tends to be "sticky" on its outside surface and will attach to other adjacent segments of intestine, to surrounding organs, or to the inner surface of the abdominal wall.

When a fistula forms between two segments of intestine, there may be no obvious bad consequences, but it is possible that the fistula can result in ingested food bypassing large segments of the intestine. This can cause decreased absorption of nutrients, leading to weight loss and malnutrition. Fistulas can pass from the intestines to adjacent organs, such as the bladder, which, in turn, leads to recurrent urinary infections.

Perianal Fistulas

The most common type of fistula occurs in the area around the anus. These anal fistulas are thought to arise from an infection or inflammation in the glands just below the lining of the anal opening. The infection or inflammation can burrow in various directions through the surrounding tissues and eventually open onto the skin in the area outside the anus. These types of fistulas, also called perianal fistulas or perineal fistulas, can be extremely distressing, and, for some individuals, dominate all other manifestations of their Crohn's disease.

Pain and Shame

When a fistula goes from the intestine to the skin of the abdominal wall or around the anus, intestinal fluid or stool comes out through the opening of the fistula on the skin. In addition to being unsightly, this intestinal fluid makes it difficult to keep the area clean and can be irritating to the surrounding skin.

Because of the location of some fistulas, they can also get in the way of some types of sexual activity. This is not simply a result of the pain that may be associated with a fistula, but also of the potential embarrassment or shame of being "unclean." If you have these feelings, it is important to realize that you are not alone. Discussing your concerns with your partner will often help soothe some of your fears and concerns about being intimate. Together, you may even be able to come up with sexual activities or positions that you both find pleasurable and that you will not find painful or uncomfortable.

People with perianal fistulas can have ongoing episodes of pain around the area of the anus, along with swelling and drainage of mucus, pus, blood, and stool. In women, the inflammation and fistulas can extend from the area around the anus to the area of the vagina. When they are particularly severe, the symptoms related to fistulas can interfere with everyday activities, such as sitting, walking, exercising, and riding a bike.

Extra-intestinal Manifestations

Both Crohn's disease and ulcerative colitis may be associated with inflammation of tissues outside of the intestinal tract, specifically the joints, eyes, skin, and liver. The extra-intestinal manifestations often occur when the intestinal disease is more active or symptomatic, but they can also occur when the bowels are not giving any trouble at all. Unfortunately, there is no good way to predict who might get these particular complications, nor do we know how to prevent them from occurring.

Joint Inflammation

Joint symptoms are probably the most common extra-intestinal manifestation of IBD, occurring in up to 30% of patients. The joints that are most commonly affected are the knees, ankles, wrists, and small joints in the fingers (knuckles) and toes. Symptoms of joint involvement or inflammation include pain and stiffness in the joints or, when severe, swelling and redness.

Sacroiliitis

A specific type of arthritis, called sacroiliitis, can occur in the lower back of patients in both Crohn's disease and ulcerative colitis. This typically presents first with stiffness in the lower back in the mornings and a vague discomfort over the lower back or hips. In a more severe form, called ankylosing spondylitis, the inflammation can extend up the spine, ultimately causing the bones of the spine to fuse together, thereby reducing flexibility and mobility. For ankylosing spondylitis, there is a blood test that can predict who is at risk for developing it but, unfortunately there is really no way to prevent its development.

Eye Inflammation

Eye inflammation is a relatively uncommon, but potentially serious, occurrence in IBD. There are several different, though closely related, forms of eye inflammation that can occur (called iritis, uveitis, and episcleritis), which all lead to red and often painful eyes. In some instances, the pain is made worse by bright lights, and there may also be blurring of vision. Any of

---

Complications of IBD Outside the Intestine (Extra-intestinal Manifestations)

- Joint symptoms (pain, stiffness, swelling)
- Sacroiliitis
- Eye inflammation
- Skin lesions
- Liver disease (primary sclerosing cholangitis)
- Bone disease

Compounded Problems

Unfortunately, some of these joint problems, particularly sacroiliitis, tend to persist even when the underlying bowel disease is adequately treated and controlled. To compound the problem, some of the drugs commonly used to treat joint inflammation, such as non-steroidal anti-inflammatory drugs, may be harmful to the intestinal tract of patients with IBD.

---

these symptoms should be assessed promptly by a doctor and treatment started. The usual treatment is medicated eyedrops containing steroids, but these should only be used after a proper examination by a qualified practitioner.

Skin Lesions

There are two main types of skin lesions that can be seen occasionally, but not frequently, in patients with IBD: erythema nodosum and pyoderma gangrenosum. Although it isn't known for certain if early treatment of the skin lesions of IBD result in better outcomes, it is important to be aware of any skin lesion that is particularly painful or enlarging for no apparent reason.

Erythema nodosum

The lesions of erythema nodosum are red or purplish, raised, and painful. They occur most often on the shins. They typically appear when the bowel symptoms are more active and go away as the bowel disease responds to treatment, sometimes leaving a small area of discoloration.

Pyoderma gangrenosum

Pyoderma gangrenosum is an area of ulcerated skin that usually occurs on the legs, but can occur on other areas of the body, particularly near the site of an ileostomy or colostomy. The lesion is sometimes painful, but it often looks much worse than it feels. The ulcerated area can grow to be quite large — sometimes 2 inches (5 cm) or even more across — and fluid can often ooze from its surface. Although it may improve when the bowel disease is treated, it does not always. When the lesions heal, they may leave areas of scarring or changed pigmentation.

Infliximab (Remicade) and adalimumab (Humira), two of the anti-tumor necrosis factor (anti-TNF) based treatments that are used to treat IBD, can be effective at healing pyoderma

---

Enlarging Lesions

- Patients often say that erythema nodosum and pyoderma gangrenosum lesions seem to start with what they thought was a bruise or an insect bite but quickly enlarge and worsen. When this happens, a doctor should be notified promptly.
- The drug infliximab (Remicade), a relatively new treatment for IBD, has been shown to be particularly effective at healing pyoderma gangrenosum lesions.

Skin Rashes

Although infliximab and adalimumab may be effective at treating the skin lesions associated with IBD, their use may also result in unusual skin rashes. These are generally not serious and can usually be managed with creams or ointments applied to the site of the rash. In rare cases, these drugs can be associated with new onset of a skin condition called psoriasis or, in some cases, a worsening of psoriasis that was present prior to the start of therapy. This is an unusual reaction to therapy because these drugs are usually quite effective at treating psoriasis.

gangrenosum lesions. When the lesions heal, they may leave areas of scarring or changed pigmentation. Although it isn't known for certain whether earlier treatment of the skin lesions of IBD result in better outcomes with treatment, it is important to be aware of any skin lesion that is particularly painful or enlarging for no apparent reason. Patients often say that erythema nodosum and pyoderma gangrenosum lesions seem to start off as what they thought was a bruise or an insect bite but quickly enlarge and worsen. When this happens, see your doctor promptly.

Liver

The most serious liver condition related to IBD is called primary sclerosing cholangitis (PSC). PSC appears to be more common in ulcerative colitis than in Crohn's disease, especially if the large intestine (colon) is involved or inflamed. PSC is thought to begin as an inflammation that specifically involves the small channels (ducts) carrying bile from the liver to the small intestine. It can lead to scarring and narrowing of these bile ducts, and, when severe or advanced, can result in damage to the liver. If the condition continues to progress, it can lead to liver cirrhosis and liver failure. PSC also predisposes the patient to episodes of bacterial infection of the bile ducts.

PSC is usually first suspected because of abnormal blood tests. This usually requires further tests or scans to see if the strictures characteristic of PSC are present. Occasionally, a liver biopsy may be necessary to sort out the possible causes. Most doctors will include blood tests of liver function and inflammation as a part of the routine checkup, even for individuals whose IBD is quite stable and not flaring. This may allow for earlier detection of PSC, but there is not an effective therapy that will prevent the progression of PSC to liver cirrhosis.

Mildly abnormal blood tests indicating liver inflammation or irritation are usually temporary and do not indicate any serious damage or long-term consequence to the liver. The abnormal blood tests are probably due to small areas of inflammation within the liver tissue that are a reaction to the associated bowel inflammation. It is not known how or why this occurs, but it tends to go away on its own and can recur repeatedly over time.

PSC is also associated with an increased risk of colorectal cancer.

Bone Disease

Although bone disease is not, strictly speaking, considered to be an extra-intestinal manifestation of the IBD, individuals

PSC Incidence

No more than 5% of people with IBD are affected by the serious liver complication called primary sclerosing cholangitis (PSC). If the condition continues to progress, it can lead to liver cirrhosis and liver failure.

Fever and Jaundice

In someone who has PSC, any episode of fever, particularly if it occurs with jaundice (yellow color) of the skin or eyes, needs to be assessed and treated immediately.

Minerals and Vitamins

For patients with IBD, maintaining an adequate intake of minerals and vitamins is an important means of preventing osteoporosis, not only good calcium and vitamin D intake but also good overall nutritional intake in terms of total calories and protein in the diet.

with IBD are at higher risk of developing certain types of bone disease. In the past, osteomalacia and rickets — serious problems with bone formation — were seen as a result of severe vitamin D deficiency in patients with Crohn's disease. These conditions are seldom seen now, probably as a result of better medical and nutritional treatments for patients with IBD.

Osteoporosis

Osteoporosis has been recognized as a prevalent condition. Osteoporosis involves a decrease in the density of the bone that occurs as a result of a reduction in the amount of minerals, such as calcium, in the bones. The bones are not strong and, therefore, susceptible to fracture with only minor trauma or sometimes without any apparent reason. Osteoporosis does not produce any symptoms until a fracture occurs.

While osteoporosis commonly occurs in older individuals without IBD, particularly in women, it seems to occur at an earlier age in patients with IBD. There are several reasons why IBD patients are more susceptible to developing osteoporosis at a younger age. The disease itself, particularly in Crohn's disease, and the associated inflammation appear to lead to reduced bone density, probably as a result of factors released into the bloodstream from the inflamed tissues. These factors, in turn, interfere with bone formation. Poor intake or absorption of certain key nutrients, such as calcium and vitamin D, may also play an important role in some patients. In addition, a person's overall nutritional state, as reflected by body weight, is also an important factor in determining bone density. In general, individuals who are underweight or malnourished tend to be more at risk of developing osteoporosis.

Medications

Medications are a major factor in the development of osteoporosis in IBD patients. In particular, steroid medications, such as prednisone, have been associated with an increased risk. Most doctors try to limit the duration of steroid treatment in their patients with IBD, and when starting someone on steroids, they will often recommend calcium and vitamin D supplements or start the patient on bisphosphonate medications (for example, etidronate, alendronate, zoledronate, and risedronate) that can help prevent further bone density loss. Most other medications used to treat IBD do not affect bone density.

The treatment of low bone density in children and adolescents with IBD is somewhat different than in adults. The period during adolescence and early adult life is critical in determining the health of the skeleton and bones in later

Osteoporosis Risk

People with IBD are at increased risk of developing osteoporosis, particularly if they have Crohn's disease or if they have received steroid medications. Some studies have indicated rates of osteoporosis of 30% in IBD patients. Osteoporosis appears to be more common in Crohn's disease than ulcerative colitis.

Bone Density Tests

Most IBD patients, particularly those with Crohn's disease, should have their bone density measured and, if it is lower than normal, it should be checked periodically (every 1 to 2 years). Bone density is measured using a safe and easy test called a DEXA (dual energy X-ray absorptiometry) that doesn't require any injections.

It has been estimated
that people with ulcerative
colitis have a 10% to 15%
risk of developing colorectal
cancer during their lifetime.

life. People reach their maximum bone density in early adulthood. However, adolescents with IBD may not be able to reach their potential maximum bone density because of poor nutritional intake, because of the underlying IBD, or because of medications. Special attention needs to be paid to adequately treating the IBD, to maintaining good nutrition, and to minimizing use of steroids during these critical years.

Cancer

While people with IBD have an increased risk of cancer, this should not be a cause for undue concern.

Cancer is a common disease that can occur in many forms and degrees of seriousness. The increased risk of cancer in IBD patients appears to be limited to one or — at most — a handful of cancer types. Risk of colorectal cancer (cancer of the rectum or large intestine) appears to be most increased in individuals with IBD.

Some recent research has suggested that patients with more inflammation occurring over a period of many years are at increased risk, but colorectal cancers can also be found in people who have had a very mild IBD course.

Q What can I do to reduce my risk of developing colorectal cancer now that I have IBD?

A The first thing to do is to determine your degree of risk. This should be done in consultation with your doctor. If it is determined that you are at increased risk, by virtue of the risk factors, then it is possible that your doctor will recommend that you should enter into a screening program. Even if screening is not recommended, regular follow-up with your doctor is important.

You may have heard of colorectal cancer screening for individuals who do not have IBD. This is different from the screening that an IBD patient would require. Some of the methods of screening used for non-IBD individuals, such as testing the stool for microscopic traces of blood, are not effective for screening IBD patients. Monitoring for symptoms of cancer is not effective because the symptoms of colorectal cancer may be very similar to those of IBD. The screening that is carried out in IBD patients involves conducting a colonoscopy in order to take numerous random biopsy samples of the colonic lining. Although this type of screening program does appear to reduce cancer rates and result in cancers being detected earlier at curable stages, it is still not a perfect method.

In recent years, efforts have been made to detect precancerous changes by using newer colonoscopy technologies so that the areas of potential concern are made visible to the naked eye, allowing biopsies specifically targeted to those areas rather than the random biopsies that have been traditionally performed.

While not everyone with IBD is at increased risk of developing colorectal cancer, it is important to be aware of the factors that do seem to increase the risk. For many years, only individuals with ulcerative colitis were considered to have an increased risk of colorectal cancer, but it now appears that people with Crohn's disease, where the large intestine is extensively affected, are also at increased risk. However, in those individuals with ulcerative colitis, where the disease is limited to the rectum and the last part of the colon, there is no significant increase in the risk of cancer. Patients diagnosed before 20 years of age, with more than an 8-year history of IBD or with associated primary sclerosing cholangitis, are at increased risk of colorectal cancer. The risk appears to increase further the longer one has had the disease. Patients with a family history of colorectal cancer involving a parent, brother, or sister are likely also at increased risk. Whether or not the severity of the IBD affects the cancer risk is not entirely known.

Risk Factors for Colorectal Cancer
• Extensive inflammation of the colon (ulcerative colitis or Crohn's colitis)
• Early age of diagnosis (less than 20 years of age)
• Long duration of disease (more than 8 years)
• Active disease symptoms
• Family history of colorectal cancer
• Primary sclerosing cholangitis (PSC)

Dysplasia

Biopsies are carefully examined by a pathologist looking for precancerous changes called dysplasia. If these changes are found, they indicate a higher possibility (10% to 20%) that the patient may already have cancer or, if cancer isn't already present, the patient has a substantial chance of developing cancer over the subsequent few years. When dysplasia is found and confirmed, surgery to remove the colon is usually recommended.

Prevention and Treatment

Because we cannot yet predict with certainty who will suffer from inflammatory bowel disease and because the causes of this disease have not yet been determined conclusively, it is difficult to recommend effective prevention strategies. The best strategy for now is to learn how to recognize the symptoms of the disease and bring them to the attention of your doctor for immediate diagnosis and treatment. In the next chapter, we present a discussion of the symptoms of inflammatory bowel disease and the tests used by doctors to diagnose this condition.

CHAPTER 2

How Do I Know I Have IBD?

CASE STUDY Jonathan

Jonathan is a 33-year-old police officer who has had several episodes of belly pain every 6 to 9 months during the past 5 years. Each time, these last between 2 and 6 weeks. Usually, the pain is crampy and tends to occur anywhere from 30 to 90 minutes after he eats. He feels bloated and uncomfortable. Jonathan also experiences watery diarrhea up to eight times a day during the pain episodes. The episodes subside on their own.

When the episodes occur, Jonathan's appetite is poor, and he can lose up to 10 pounds. In between the episodes, he has no pain and regains most of the weight that he lost. However, during the past 2 years, he has felt more tired than usual.

Jonathan doesn't think much of these episodes. His wife has irritable bowel syndrome, a condition she has been told is related to diet and stress, and he figures that he has something similar. However, this year, Jonathan happens to have had his annual physical examination shortly after an episode of pain and diarrhea, and he mentions it in passing to his doctor.

After further questioning, his doctor is concerned that Jonathan may be suffering from something more serious than irritable bowel syndrome. He is concerned about the weight loss that occurs during the episodes and the fact that Jonathan wakes up from his sleep with pain and diarrhea. In addition, the doctor is able to feel a tender area of swelling in the lower right area of Jonathan's abdomen.

Based upon these findings, the doctor is concerned that Jonathan may have Crohn's disease in the ileum (the last part of the small intestine). He decides to order tests to investigate further…

(continued on page 148)

Recognizing Symptoms

Sometimes, people, particularly young people, delay seeking medical attention for inflammatory bowel disease because they believe that they will remain healthy and that any symptoms they experience are likely due to simple conditions that are probably not long-lasting. Although some people feel that the symptoms are suspicious, they may deny the possibility of having a serious chronic disease, especially if they already have a family history of IBD and do not wish to face the possibility that they, too, are going to have to live with this disease. In some cases, the delay in diagnosis may be due to a general lack of knowledge on the part of the individual about what constitutes abnormal or unacceptable symptoms or due to embarrassment that they may feel in discussing their symptoms. Very occasionally, a delay in diagnosis may occur when a physician discounts a patient's description of symptoms or misses important clinical clues toward making the diagnosis.

For most people, any delay between the time symptoms begin and the time they ask their doctor for advice is due to the gradual change from a state of good health to a state of illness or disease. There are likely very few individuals with IBD who do not eventually undergo evaluation and have a diagnosis of Crohn's disease or ulcerative colitis confirmed.

> **Good Health**
>
> Crohn's disease and ulcerative colitis typically develop in people who previously were in good health and who had no prior bowel symptoms or digestive problems.

Common Symptoms

Inflammatory bowel disease, in particular, Crohn's disease, can present with quite different symptoms from one person to the next, and these symptoms depend upon many different factors.

Some factors are not directly related to the disease. These include usual bowel habits before developing IBD, pain tolerance or threshold, and probably even mood. Although these individual factors may modify the symptom experience, the nature of the inflammation — its severity, extent, and location — is most important in determining the symptoms.

Crohn's disease and ulcerative colitis tend to share a number of symptoms, such as abdominal pain and diarrhea, but they can be quite different with respect to the prominence of these symptoms and their course over time. Listed below are the common symptoms of the two disorders and how they manifest.

> **Flare Periods**
>
> Crohn's disease and ulcerative colitis fluctuate in severity, and patients can experience flares and remissions. Symptoms are typically experienced primarily during these flare periods. When the disease is in remission, patients, particularly patients with ulcerative colitis, may have no symptoms whatsoever.

Ulcerative Colitis Symptoms

Because ulcerative colitis affects only the large intestine, the symptoms are due to inflammation, damage, and ulceration of the lining of the large intestine. The inflammation is usually contained within the most superficial inner linings of the large intestine. This determines the type of symptoms that a patient may experience. Because of these symptoms, patients with ulcerative colitis often feel they have to stay close to a bathroom when their disease is active.

Blood in the Stool

The most obvious and consistent manifestation of ulcerative colitis is the presence of blood in the stool. This occurs in almost every individual with ulcerative colitis. In fact, if someone with IBD has never had blood in the stools, it is quite possible that the condition is Crohn's disease rather than ulcerative colitis. Crohn's disease is not always associated with blood in the stool.

Rectal Bleeding

Inflammation of the rectum always occurs in ulcerative colitis and affects the normal ability to hold stool and gas.

Blood in the stool occurs regardless of whether the inflammation is restricted to just the bottom end of the large intestine (rectum) or involves the entire large intestine. In some cases, blood and mucus may be passed without any stool. Although this bleeding can happen with every bowel movement and can appear quite severe, it almost never results in a sudden fall in the hemoglobin (blood count), and, as a result, the bleeding is almost never an emergency situation. It is, however, an indication of the severity of the underlying inflammation and requires medical attention.

Other common conditions, such as hemorrhoids, can also cause blood with stools, so not all rectal bleeding is due to ulcerative colitis. In ulcerative colitis, mucus is frequently passed along with blood.

Rectal Urgency

Inflammation of the rectum always occurs in ulcerative colitis and affects the normal ability to hold stool and gas. Patients with ulcerative colitis may experience frequent and very strong urges to move the bowels whenever there is the smallest amount of stool, blood, mucus, or gas in the rectum. This urgency is often accompanied by strong lower abdominal cramping that is probably due to contraction or spasm of the rectum and sigmoid colon.

When patients experience this type of urgency and are not close to a bathroom, they may not be able to control the urge long enough and may be incontinent. This loss of control can sometimes be the most troubling symptom for patients with ulcerative colitis. In many cases, individuals with active ulcerative colitis will plan their activities so that they always have easy and quick access to a bathroom.

The increased bowel activity usually occurs in the early morning hours and soon after eating. As a result, patients will avoid going out in the morning until after bowel movements subside, or they will avoid eating before going out of the house. When the ulcerative colitis is more severe, the bowel activity may continue throughout the night and will make the patient wake up several times to go to the bathroom.

Abdominal Pain

The inflammation of the inner lining of the intestine can produce abdominal pain, but because the inner lining of the intestine does not have nerve endings that can detect painful stimuli, abdominal pain is not a constant feature in most cases of ulcerative colitis. When it does occur, pain tends to be crampy, occurring around the time of bowel movements, and is often associated with rectal urgency. This pain is probably due more to the contraction or spasm of the intestine than to the inflammation of the inner lining itself.

> **Unrelenting Pain**
>
> Between flares, patients usually do not feel any pain. If a patient with ulcerative colitis reports constant, unrelenting abdominal pain, it suggests the possibility of another diagnosis or a complication, such as bowel perforation. Be sure to consult with your doctor if abdominal pain has this characteristic.

False Urges

False urges are another troubling symptom that many patients with active ulcerative colitis experience. When the rectum becomes distended with gas or stool, it sends a signal to the brain indicating a need to move one's bowels. When the rectum is inflamed, it becomes irritable and will send these signals to the brain with only the smallest amount of distension or even without any distension at all.

In that case, a person will feel a strong urge to move the bowels and will rush to the bathroom, only to find that nothing comes out or, at most, just a small amount of blood and mucus. As a result, people with ulcerative colitis may have to make countless trips to the bathroom every day, even though they may pass stool only a handful of times.

Typically, when stool is passed, it comes in only small amounts each time. Because patients will pass what is recognized as stool only very infrequently, they will sometimes feel as if they are constipated. When only the rectum is inflamed, the inflammation and spasm may actually block the normal stool that is present in the large intestine above the rectum from getting through and being excreted.

Diarrhea

When the inflammation of the large intestine extends above the rectum, it affects the normal fluid absorptive function of the large intestine, resulting in loose or liquid stools, also known as diarrhea. The liquid stool may be mixed with variable amounts of blood and mucus.

Intestinal Gas

Some patients experiencing a flare of ulcerative colitis will feel that they have an increased amount of gas or that the odor of the gas changes. Some even say that they can tell when a flare is about to come on because of this change in the odor. The amount of gas produced during a flare of colitis has never actually been studied, but it is likely that, even if the amount of gas produced is not increased, the inflamed rectum and large intestine are more sensitive to the presence of gas and, therefore, will pass it more frequently.

Fatigue

When the inflammation in the colon is particularly bad or when it involves a large portion of the colon, patients with ulcerative colitis may suffer from fatigue and weight loss. The fatigue is most often due to the inflammation itself, but can also be due to anemia resulting from blood loss in the stool. Chronic blood loss can, over time, lead to iron deficiency anemia. When a person is anemic, the blood is not able to carry oxygen to the tissues in the body as effectively, and, as a result, a person may experience fatigue and breathlessness with minimal amounts of exertion.

Weight Loss

Cytokines can also produce changes in metabolism that result in loss of body weight, even when food intake is at a level that should be sufficient to maintain a person's healthy nutritional state.

Cytokines
Intestinal inflammation itself, even without producing anemia or iron deficiency, can also produce fatigue. This probably occurs as a result of certain proteins, called cytokines, that are released from inflamed tissues and that can produce symptoms such as fatigue, loss of appetite, and fever.

Crohn's Disease Symptoms

Crohn's disease can affect any part of the gastrointestinal tract. As a result, the symptoms reported by patients with Crohn's disease can be much more varied than those reported by patients with ulcerative colitis.

As with ulcerative colitis, the symptoms experienced in Crohn's disease are highly dependent upon the location and severity of the inflammation within the gastrointestinal tract. However, the relative prominence of the symptoms may be different in Crohn's disease than in ulcerative colitis. Because there are locations that are much more commonly affected than others, there are presenting symptoms that also tend to be more common than others. As a general rule, abdominal pain, diarrhea, fatigue, and weight loss tend to be the most common presenting symptoms in Crohn's disease. In children, failure to grow normally, or "failure to thrive," is a common presenting symptom.

Atypical Symptoms

Because the locations within the gut that are affected by the disease vary from person to person, there is no "typical" patient or "typical" symptom presentation in Crohn's disease.

Quick Guide to Crohn's Disease Symptoms

The symptoms of Crohn's disease are similar to the symptoms of ulcerative colitis. However, a number of additional symptoms, not typically experienced in ulcerative colitis, may be experienced in patients with Crohn's disease. One problem that is very uncommon in ulcerative colitis, but may be seen in Crohn's disease, is the occurrence of fistulas and abscesses around the anus and ulcers within the anal canal. These complications occur because of the tendency of Crohn's disease to penetrate more deeply into the bowel lining.

If you should experience any one or combination of the following symptoms, be sure to consult with your doctor.

- Rectal bleeding (blood and mucus in the stool)
- Rectal urgency (frequent trips to the toilet and urgent need to move the bowels that often can't be delayed)
- Severe abdominal cramps
- Frequent diarrhea
- Increased intestinal gas
- Persistent fatigue
- Weight loss
- Fistulas and abscesses around the anus and ulcers within the anal canal
- Failure to grow or thrive in children

Tips for Working with Your Doctor

Working with your doctor to diagnose your symptoms is the first step in understanding and treating inflammatory bowel disease. However, some patients find their initial meeting with their doctor somewhat unsatisfactory because they do not have enough time to ask all the questions they may have. While most doctors do have busy schedules, you can make the most of your appointments with them by being well prepared. To get the most out of your visit to your doctor, try the following tips:

Make sure there is enough time.

If you think that your problems and concerns are going to take longer than the time your doctor usually allocates for an appointment, ask for a longer meeting. You will find this much more satisfactory than trying to "find a moment" at the end of the appointment to raise what may be your most pressing questions and concerns. If you do come to the end of your allotted time, acknowledge to the doctor that you have run out of time and that you still have items to discuss. The doctor may sometimes ask you to continue or, in some cases, suggest that you schedule another appointment.

Keep your description of symptoms focused and factual.

The doctor wants to hear about what you are feeling, so just describe what you are experiencing without jumping to conclusions or making speculations. You might say to your doctor, "I'm here today because I keep getting episodes when I can't move my bowels, my belly becomes distended like I'm 9 months pregnant, and I start vomiting. It feels exactly like it did when I had surgery for a bowel obstruction 4 years ago, but maybe a little less severe." Although you may suspect this is caused by a bowel obstruction, you don't need to interpret the experience or make a diagnosis. That is the doctor's job — to determine if the symptoms are due to a bowel obstruction or due to some other cause or condition that could produce similar symptoms.

Bring a list of your medications and their doses.

The doctor will need to know if you are taking any medications and their dosage. Report if you have experienced any side effects and when they first started in relation to when you began taking the medications.

Make a list of your questions and issues.

Keep your list of questions short enough that it can be covered in the available time and try to make sure that the questions are specific and to the point rather than being overly general and difficult to answer concisely. For example, answering a question such as "What are the possible side effects of this medication?" may take up the entire appointment, whereas asking "What are the common and serious side effects of this drug?" will get the information you are really looking for in a relatively short time, allowing time for other questions.

Prioritize your list of questions from most important to the least important.

Take care of the questions that are causing you the most concern first so that you can feel more at ease and more comfortable asking other questions. Often your doctor's answer to the most pressing question also answers other questions on your list.

Bring a friend or relative to help you remember what you have discussed.

Many patients ask a spouse, relative, or friend to accompany them to the appointment, to help them remember the questions they planned to ask and make note of the answers given by the doctor. Their emotional support is also important.

Make notes about key points in the discussion.

You or your companion should make a record of what your doctor investigates and concludes so that you can follow any treatment program the doctor may prescribe. This is especially important if treatment options are presented to you for your decision. You may want to refer to your notes when making your decision.

Abdominal Pain

Unlike ulcerative colitis, where the inflammation is limited to the innermost lining of the intestine, in Crohn's disease the inflammation and ulcers can penetrate through all the layers of the intestinal wall. Since there are nerves that can transmit pain signals in the deeper layers of the intestine, this means that pain may be a more consistent feature of Crohn's disease.

Strictures and Blockages

Immediate Medical Attention

Episodes of abdominal pain that last more than 4 to 6 hours without passage of gas or stool require immediate medical attention and often require hospitalization.

If Crohn's disease produces some narrowing of the intestine (most often in the small intestine), it can produce some degree of blockage, making it difficult for food and intestinal contents to get through the narrowed areas. This can be experienced as crampy abdominal pain that occurs within minutes to several hours after a meal, depending on the precise location of the narrowing. Bloating of the abdomen can occur along with this pain, and, when it is particularly severe, nausea and vomiting may also occur. More complete blockages can occur, and these will be associated with symptoms of abdominal pain, distension, nausea, and vomiting. During the episode, the person may not be able to pass any stool or gas.

Bowel Movements

As is the case in ulcerative colitis, patients with Crohn's disease may have crampy abdominal pain around the time of bowel movements. This may be due to irritability of the intestine and the associated spasm that can occur as a result of inflammation.

Diarrhea

Diarrhea is a common, but not universal, symptom of Crohn's disease. In fact, some patients with intestinal narrowing actually present with decreased bowel movements and constipation. The diarrhea that occurs in patients with Crohn's disease is usually not bloody, but when the lower part of the large intestine is inflamed, bleeding can occur more often.

Fatigue

Fatigue is a very common symptom in Crohn's disease and can be one of the most difficult symptoms to completely reverse with medical therapy. As in ulcerative colitis, it is probably due to the release of cytokines from the inflamed intestinal tissues.

Weight Loss

Weight loss may be due to the changes in metabolism caused by the cytokines, but it can also be caused by reduced nutrient intake as a result of pain that occurs after eating. In patients with small intestinal inflammation, there may be problems with absorption of nutrients, which can lead to weight loss.

Anal Problems

While patients with ulcerative colitis may describe irritation of the skin around the anus or may even develop hemorrhoids (swollen veins) because of the frequent bowel movements, patients with Crohn's disease are at risk of developing certain specific problems that are more serious. They can develop anal fissures or ulcers (painful breaks in the skin inside the anus), abscesses (painful collections of pus), and fistulas (small openings to the skin around the anus that can drain stool, pus, or blood).

Extra-intestinal Symptoms

Both ulcerative colitis and Crohn's disease can present with certain associated symptoms or conditions outside of the intestine. These are called extra-intestinal manifestations and are usually due to inflammation of other tissues outside of the bowel — joints, eyes, skin, and liver, for example. Joint manifestations (arthritis) are the most common. These extra-intestinal manifestations can occur at the time of first diagnosis of IBD, or they can occur later on in the course of the disease. In occasional cases, they can first occur months or even years before the bowel symptoms first become apparent. The same major extra-intestinal manifestations and symptoms (joint, eye, skin, and liver) can occur in both disorders.

> **Nutrient Deficiencies**
>
> Depending on the part of the intestine involved in Crohn's disease, patients can develop specific nutrient deficiencies. For example, the last part of the small intestine (terminal ileum) is commonly affected in Crohn's disease; this is also where vitamin B_{12} is absorbed. As a result, vitamin B_{12} deficiency can develop in patients with Crohn's disease of the terminal ileum.

Onset of Symptoms

Inflammatory bowel disease usually first develops in one of three different patterns of symptom onset: gradual, sudden, and relapsing or remitting.

Gradual Onset

Most often, Crohn's disease and ulcerative colitis develop very gradually so that it takes many weeks, months, or, in some cases, years before patients recognize the symptoms and mention them to their doctor for diagnosis.

Sudden Onset

Unusually, though certainly not rarely, inflammatory bowel disease develops abruptly. Symptoms may come on suddenly, sometimes so quickly that the disease seems to develop virtually overnight, with the person going from a state of good health to a serious and severe illness without any obvious warning. This type of presentation is quite striking and can often make it very difficult for patients and their families. Important medical management decisions, including the choice of medications and the possibility of undergoing surgery, may be required.

Relapsing or Remitting Onset

Inflammatory bowel disease may also develop following a so-called relapsing or remitting course. Patients can present with mild episodes or flares that occur for days, weeks, or even months at a time. During these flares, symptoms get noticeably worse, but then seem to go away spontaneously (also called "going into remission") so that the person goes back to a state of normal health with no symptoms for many weeks, months, or even years before another episode or flare occurs.

Because these flares often subside on their own, patients will sometimes not go to the doctor for investigation or treatment, until an episode is more severe, lasts longer than usual, or is more concerning in some way.

Diagnostic Tests for IBD

- Blood tests
- Stool tests
- Imaging studies
  - X-ray
  - Ultrasound
  - CT scan
  - MRI
  - Nuclear medicine Labeled WBC imaging
- Endoscopy
  - Gastroscopy
  - Colonoscopy
  - Wireless capsule Endoscopy
- Biopsy

Diagnostic Methods

If you suspect you or a family member is experiencing any symptoms of inflammatory bowel disease, be sure to see your doctor as soon as possible. A medical history of symptoms and a physical examination are usually adequate for strongly suspecting a diagnosis of Crohn's disease and ulcerative colitis, but further diagnostic testing is important in confirming the suspected diagnosis, determining the extent and severity of the disease, and screening for possible complications of the disease. These procedures include standard blood and stool tests, various imaging studies, endoscopies, and biopsy.

Not all tests or investigations are required in all patients. The tests chosen will depend on your specific symptoms, as well as the availability, potential risk, and discomfort of the specific investigation.

Blood Tests

White blood cell or platelet count can be elevated in active IBD. Certain antibodies are found more frequently in the blood of patients with IBD. Antibodies are proteins produced by the immune system to defend against certain types of infection by binding to specific molecules found on the surface of viruses and bacteria. Some proteins, most commonly, C-reactive protein, are found in higher levels in the blood of people with inflammatory conditions.

Antibody Patterns

The pattern of antibodies may help differentiate between ulcerative colitis and Crohn's disease. One of these antibodies, called perinuclear antineutrophil cytoplasmic antibody (pANCA), occurs more commonly in ulcerative colitis, whereas another antibody, anti-Saccharomyces cerevisiae antibody (ASCA), is fairly specific for Crohn's disease.

There are several other antibody tests that are commercially available along with pANCA and ASCA. Although this panel of antibody tests cannot replace more definitive diagnostic tests, such as X-rays, endoscopy, or biopsy, and although they cannot yet be used to confirm a diagnosis of IBD, they may be helpful in screening out patients with possible IBD before proceeding to more definitive and often invasive diagnostic testing. This may be particularly helpful in children, where invasive diagnostic testing is more difficult to justify and carry out, particularly when the suspicion of actually finding disease is relatively low. These antibody tests can be used to help determine who should undergo further testing, since it is very unlikely that a child with a negative pANCA and ASCA test will turn out to have IBD. It also appears that, in a patient with known Crohn's disease or ulcerative colitis, certain patterns of the different antibodies, and the levels of antibodies present in the blood, may be associated with certain disease locations and with higher risk of developing certain complications of disease.

Other blood tests indicate evidence of possible complications or nutritional deficiencies that may have

Screening
Although blood tests cannot replace more definitive diagnostic tests, such as X-rays, endoscopy, or biopsy, and although they cannot yet be used to confirm a diagnosis, they may be helpful in screening out patients with possible IBD before proceeding to more definitive and often invasive diagnostic testing.

occurred as a result of IBD. These include anemia, liver disease, iron deficiency, vitamin B_{12} deficiency, and calcium deficiency.

Stool Tests

Stool samples may be sent for culture to rule out a bacterial infection as the cause for a patient's symptoms. While the yield from this is quite low, particularly when symptoms have been going on for many weeks or even months, it is important to rule out infections before embarking on many types of therapy for Crohn's disease and ulcerative colitis.

Stool may also be examined for parasites or the eggs of parasites. Occasionally, the laboratory will report that no parasites were seen, but that many white blood cells are present in the stool. The presence of white blood cells almost always indicates some type of inflammatory condition in the intestine. Stool can also be tested for certain proteins — calprotectin and lactoferrin — that are present in white blood cells that indicate the presence of active intestinal inflammation.

Disease Activity

Stool tests can be used to monitor disease activity and response to treatment. These tests, when combined with blood tests, help make decisions regarding changes in treatment strategies.

Imaging Studies

Imaging studies provide "pictures" of the intestines and other internal organs without having to open up the abdomen by performing surgery. Imaging studies have been the mainstay of IBD diagnosis for many years. X-rays provide two-dimensional pictures of the intestine, while other types of imaging studies

X-rays

Since the intestine does not appear in sufficient detail on plain X-rays, a contrast agent, usually barium, is used to fill the intestine so that the intestinal lining and wall can be seen in contrast to the barium. The barium is administered in several ways, depending on the area of bowel under examination:

Upper GI Series and Small Bowel Follow-Through

When examining the small intestine, the barium can be given by having the person drink it. X-rays are taken every few minutes as the barium passes out of the stomach and through the small intestine. This type of X-ray can also detect problems in the esophagus, stomach, and duodenum. It requires no preparation on the part of the patient other than having to fast on the day of the examination.

Small Bowel Enema, or Enteroclysis

In some cases, a small bowel follow-through X-ray doesn't provide enough detail because of problems with the movement of barium through the small intestine or because the images are captured only every few minutes and important information can be missed. To solve this problem, the barium is administered directly into the small intestine by means of a tube placed through the nose into the esophagus, stomach, and duodenum. The radiologist can watch continuously as the barium flows through the entire small intestine. This examination also requires only fasting prior to the procedure.

Barium Enema

The upper GI series and small bowel follow-through do not provide any information about the large intestine. When imaging of the large intestine is required, the physician may order a barium enema, where a tube is inserted into the rectum and barium and air are pumped into the large intestine. The patient needs to prepare for this procedure by taking a regimen of laxatives intended to clean out all the stool from the large intestine. The barium enema is rarely performed, however, replaced by MRI studies, CT scans and colonoscopy.

X-ray Risk

All X-rays involve some degree of exposure to radiation, but, as long as the tests are not repeated frequently, the amount of radiation exposure is relatively small compared to the amount that one is exposed to every day from background sources.

also provide information about surrounding structures within the abdomen, something which conventional X-ray studies cannot do. These include ultrasounds, computer-assisted tomography (CT, or CAT) scans, and magnetic resonance imaging (MRI). They provide multiple images of the abdomen in "slices" that can be positioned crosswise or lengthwise through the abdomen. In this way, it is possible to provide a three-dimensional representation of the intestines, other abdominal organs, and even blood vessels.

Ultrasound

Ultrasound examinations are very safe and widely available. A probe that transmits a high-frequency sound wave is moved over the abdominal wall. That sound wave is reflected off structures within the abdomen and back to the probe, which has a sensor to detect the reflected sound waves, or echoes. These echoes are then converted into an image. Patients must fast before an abdominal ultrasound study.

One particular type of ultrasound, a transanal ultrasound, is used to evaluate patients for possible anal abscesses and fistulas. This involves putting a special ultrasound probe into the anus in order to obtain images of the surrounding tissues. Although this may provide excellent detail, the procedure may be very difficult or impossible for patients with painful anal conditions associated with Crohn's disease.

Computer-Assisted Tomography (CAT scan, or CT scan)

Computer-assisted tomography is a very safe and widely used imaging technique. This technology may supplant small bowel follow-through and small bowel enema procedures.

During a CT scan, the patient lies on a table, which is surrounded by a large donut-shaped structure that produces and detects X-rays. These X-rays are converted into very detailed images when processed in the machine's computer.

Patients undergoing CT scans of the abdomen are often given a contrast solution to drink 1 to 2 hours before the scan to provide better diagnostic images or an intravenous injection of another contrast material to show blood supply to the intestine and other tissues.

CT scans are generally not needed for routine follow-up of a patient's clinical disease activity. If an abscess is detected by CT scan, the images can be used by the radiologist to insert a needle or plastic tube through the skin and into the abscess in order to allow it to drain properly.

Detecting Complications

Ultrasound may be helpful in detecting complications of IBD, such as abscesses, but it is not the most sensitive imaging study, particularly when the intestines are to be evaluated.

Sensitive Test

CT scans are very sensitive at detecting IBD complications, such as abscesses and intestinal obstructions. They do involve some radiation exposure and so should not be repeated too frequently or unnecessarily.

Magnetic Resonance Imaging (MRI)

Magnetic resonance imaging is relatively new in IBD diagnosis. It uses a large magnet to create images based upon the different water content and molecular makeup of different tissues. A patient undergoing an MRI scan lies on a table that slides into the machine. The patient lies very still during the procedure, which can last up to 20 or 30 minutes. Like a CT scan, the MRI provides cross-sectional images, but because the intestines are continuously contracting in the abdomen during the procedure, the images of the intestines may not be as clear as they are in CT scans, where the image is obtained in a fraction of a second. Some studies are done after patients are administered an injection of a contrast agent into the vein. Because it does not involve any exposure to radiation, MRI may become the investigation of choice once the technology has advanced to the point where it provides images that are comparable in quality to barium X-rays and CT scans.

MRI is particularly useful for assessing the anus and the surrounding tissue for complications, such as fistulas and abscesses, in Crohn's disease. MRI is also useful in determining whether areas of the intestine are inflamed or whether the changes seen are due to scarring. This is a particularly helpful distinction because tissue that is inflamed may respond to therapy with medication, whereas areas of scarring will likely not improve with medical therapy.

> **Assessing the Anus**
>
> MRI is particularly useful for assessing the anus and the surrounding tissue for complications, such as fistulas and abscesses, in Crohn's disease.

Nuclear Medicine Labeled WBC Imaging

These various imaging methods provide very good information about the structure of the gastrointestinal tract and complications of IBD, such as fistulas or abscesses, but in the past, they have not always provided detailed information about the degree of inflammation present within the inner lining of the intestine. To show the amount of inflammatory cells (white blood cells, or WBC) within the bowel wall, nuclear medicine labeled WBC imaging is used, most commonly when the physician wishes to evaluate the small intestine in a patient with Crohn's disease.

A blood sample is first taken from the patient and then the white blood cells are tagged with a molecular marker (radio-isotope) emitting radiation that can be detected by a special imaging machine. The tagged white blood cells are then reinjected into the patient's bloodstream, and images of the abdomen are taken using the special nuclear medicine imaging machine. The areas of inflammation attract many of the tagged white blood cells, and light up on the pictures that are taken by the machine. However, areas of the intestine that may be scarred from previous attacks of IBD, but are not presently inflamed, will not show up on the images.

> **Reversing or Reducing Symptoms**
>
> The information derived from a nuclear medicine labeled WBC imaging test may help the physician decide if medical treatment will be effective in reversing or reducing symptoms. If symptoms are due to scarring without significant inflammation, it is unlikely that any medication will help.

As other imaging techniques, especially MRI, become better at detecting subtle amounts of inflammation, the use of the imaging techniques that involve exposure to radiation — for example, CT scan and labeled WBC imaging — will likely become less frequently used. It is already very rare to see WBC imaging used, and many doctors are trying to minimize the use of CT scans whenever possible.

Endoscopy

In endoscopy, a long, narrow tube with a light and a camera on its tip is passed into the gastrointestinal tract. The endoscope can be steered in the desired direction to provide very detailed images of the inner lining of the gastrointestinal tract on a television monitor. When the procedure examines the esophagus, stomach, and duodenum, it is called an upper gastrointestinal endoscopy or, more commonly, a gastroscopy. When the instrument is inserted through the anus into the rectum and colon, it is called a colonoscopy. When doing a colonoscopy, the physician can often also examine the ileum (last part of the small intestine). This is one of the areas most commonly involved in Crohn's disease.

Gastroscopy

Gastroscopy is a relatively straightforward procedure, but is done much less commonly in IBD than is colonoscopy, with the possible exception of individuals first diagnosed in childhood. In that case, gastroscopy is frequently carried out at the time of diagnosis. Gastroscopy is usually carried out following an overnight fast so that the stomach is empty. The back of the throat is sprayed with a local anesthetic so that the gag reflex is reduced, and, in some cases, a mild sedative is given intravenously to relax the patient. The whole procedure usually takes no more than 10 to 15 minutes and is typically not painful. In young children, it may be necessary to administer heavier sedation or general anesthetic in order to carry out the procedure.

Colonoscopy

Colonoscopy requires preparation of the bowel with a special diet (usually clear liquids) and a special laxative for one or more days prior to the procedure. This is important because the presence of feces can interfere with visibility and make the procedure almost useless. In some cases, the physician may not order a special laxative for the patient. Usually this is when the IBD is very active, but even in these instances a smaller or more gentle preparation is probably still advisable and safe.

Upper Gastrointestinal Endoscopy

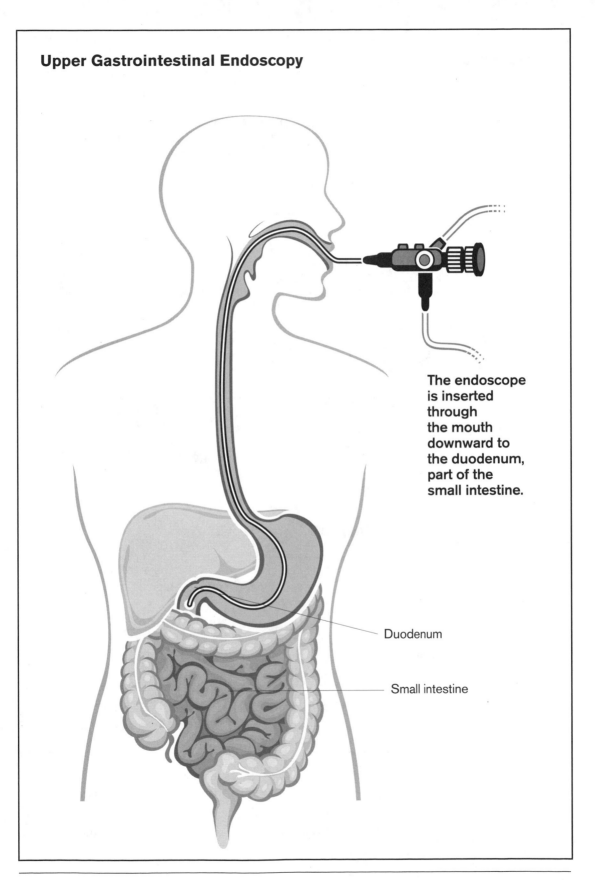

The endoscope is inserted through the mouth downward to the duodenum, part of the small intestine.

Duodenum

Small intestine

Colonoscopy

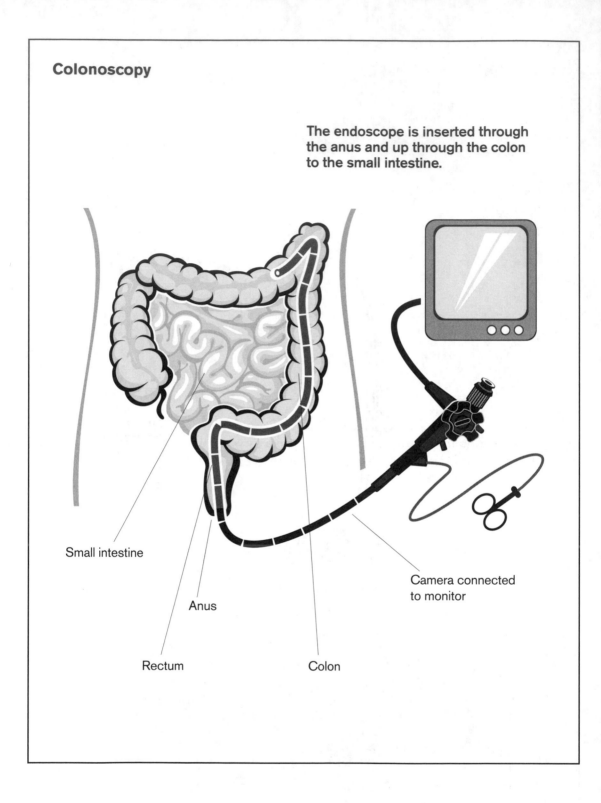

The endoscope is inserted through the anus and up through the colon to the small intestine.

Small intestine

Anus

Rectum

Colon

Camera connected to monitor

The colonoscopy procedure itself is usually performed with a sedative and an analgesic (pain medication). It typically takes 15 to 45 minutes to complete. It is generally quite a safe procedure, with a very small risk of serious complications, but some degree of abdominal pain and cramping is not unusual at times during the procedure. In most cases, the medication given before the procedure helps to minimize the discomfort.

Wireless Capsule Endoscopy

Standard gastroscopy and colonoscopy are not able to reach large segments of the small intestine that may be affected in Crohn's disease. The imaging studies that can take pictures of those areas of the small intestine are improving, but do not always provide the detailed images required by the physician to make management recommendations. Wireless capsule endoscopy (WCE), or PillCam technology, was developed to provide the types of high-quality visual images of the inner lining of the small intestine that are provided by gastroscopy in the stomach and duodenum and by colonoscopy in the colon and ileum. In most cases, the procedure allows examination of the entire length of small intestine.

A capsule — about the size of a large vitamin pill or capsule — that contains a battery, light source, and a tiny lens and camera chip is swallowed by the patient and begins taking two pictures every second during an 8-hour period. It is propelled through the esophagus, stomach, and small bowel by the normal muscular movements of the gastrointestinal tract in the same way food is passed down along the gastrointestinal tract. The patient wears a recording device, much like a cellular telephone, and can go about daily activities. Once the procedure is over, images are downloaded from the recorder to a computer. The physician can then look for signs of Crohn's disease.

Despite the fact that the WCE can provide excellent images of the entire small intestine, it is not commonly used in IBD diagnosis. In ulcerative colitis, the small intestine is not involved and does not require this type of detailed evaluation. In Crohn's disease, care must be taken because the capsule could produce a blockage or bowel obstruction in any strictures of the intestine. Nevertheless, the capsule may be helpful in diagnosing subtle degrees of Crohn's disease in the small intestine, where the other imaging techniques do not provide a full answer to the patient's symptoms.

> ### Extremely Useful
>
> Colonoscopy is an extremely useful diagnostic test in IBD. It will always detect ulcerative colitis if it is present, and will detect Crohn's disease in 80% to 90% of cases. In 10% to 20% of cases of Crohn's disease, the procedure is not able to examine the areas of disease because of technical factors or because the disease is beyond the reach of the colonoscope.

Enteroscopy

A number of innovations have been developed in the area of endoscopy to allow examination of areas of the small intestine that are beyond the reach of the standard gastroscope and colonoscope.

- Push enteroscopy uses a longer than normal gastroscope to get further into the small intestine, but the success of this procedure is limited because of the floppiness and many twists and turns of the small intestine.

- Double balloon enteroscopy (DBE) generally allows more extensive examination of the small intestine through sequential inflation and deflation of two balloons near the tip of the instrument. This inflation and deflation helps to propel the tip of the instrument along the small intestine. The technique can be performed through the mouth, esophagus, and stomach into the first part of the small intestine, or it can be performed from below through the colon into the last part of the small intestine. It tends to be a longer procedure than standard endoscopy and typically requires general anesthetic or propofol for deep sedation. Biopsies can be obtained of the inner lining of the small intestine, and the rate of progress through the small intestine is under the control of the physician, as opposed to the wireless capsule endoscopy, where the progress through the intestinal tract is largely determined by contractions of the small intestine.

Biopsies

Endoscopy also allows the operator to perform biopsies of the inner lining of the gastrointestinal tract. Small samples are taken with a tiny instrument with small jaws that can cut or pull off pieces of the inner lining. This part of the procedure is not painful; usually, the patient is not aware that it is happening. The biopsy process is very safe; complications, such as serious bleeding, are extremely uncommon.

In some instances, biopsies are done to screen for precancerous changes. Some patients with IBD involving the large intestine for more than 8 to 10 years are at increased risk of colon cancer, and their physicians may recommend a surveillance program that involves regular colonoscopy with many biopsies taken throughout the colon.

Rule Out Other Conditions

Biopsies are usually taken to confirm the suspected diagnosis of IBD and to help rule out other conditions, such as infection. As surprising as it may seem, biopsies do not always provide 100% certainty about the diagnosis, particularly when distinguishing between Crohn's disease and ulcerative colitis. Other information, such as the location of the inflammation or other associated features, provides more assistance in diagnosis.

Prognosis

Once the diagnosis of IBD has been confirmed using one or more of the available investigations, some of that information can be used to help the physician determine the severity and prognosis of a patient's particular IBD. However, even with the most complete diagnostic staging, the ultimate prognosis can be unpredictable, varying from person to person with the same disorder. Patients naturally have many pressing questions about the course of their disease, which are asked and answered in the next chapter.

CHAPTER 3

What Can I Expect Now That I Have IBD?

CASE STUDY Kelly

After asking her doctor a host of questions about the symptoms and diagnosis of ulcerative colitis, Kelly was still upset because she knows of a boy who went to her high school who had ulcerative colitis. Her recollection of him was that he was sick for many days at a time. He finally had to take several weeks off school and have surgery. She is concerned that a similar fate awaits her and that she will fall behind in her university studies — or possibly even have to drop out. Even worse, she fears she may have to wear a bag to collect her stool. She has heard that people with colitis live shorter lives and are likely to develop colon cancer.

From her doctor, Kelly wants to know if the disease will get worse. What are the chances of her getting better? Will she require surgery and need a bag to collect her stool? Will she be able to live a full, productive life — complete her studies, go to work, have a family? Can she expect to live a normal life? Can she travel? And most urgently, can she die from IBD?

Again, her doctor set out to give her the information she needed to cope with her uncertainties and anxieties. Every person with IBD is unique, he told her. Just because someone she knows had a difficult time does not mean that she necessarily will. IBD is not a fatal condition, he assured her, and the majority of individuals with IBD lead productive lives — they are able to complete their studies, go to work, and have a family.

Kelly had many more questions to ask, but for now, her doctor provided her with some links to some valuable and credible websites, while cautioning her against relying on websites from unrecognized sources and discussing her disease with others in Internet chat rooms or bulletin boards. If she ever felt concerned about the reliability of the information she was finding from any source, he welcomed her to discuss it with him.

Frequently Asked Questions

If you or a member of your family has been recently diagnosed with inflammatory bowel disease, you will likely have a number of puzzling questions, concerns, thoughts, and feelings about this condition. Different individuals have different ways of responding to bad news. For some people, there will be fear and anxiety; for others, there will be anger; for still others, there will be sadness. Some will take the news in stride, seeing the disease as a challenge, an obstacle that needs to be overcome like any other challenge they might encounter day to day. Some people will try to deny their illness or try to minimize its significance. None of these feelings or approaches to coping with disease is wrong, as long as it does not prevent the IBD sufferer from obtaining advice and care from medical professionals.

In most cases, you will know very little about the disease, which is to be expected, since most of us, unless we work in the health-care field or have a relative with IBD, may not have even heard about these disorders. You will probably want to ask a number of very specific questions, even if you already know someone with IBD or if you have learned about IBD through some other means. Ask your doctor all the questions that come to mind. The answers to common questions about the course and prognosis of IBD are addressed in this chapter.

Coping with Knowledge

One way of coping with this disease is to learn as much as possible about it. In most instances, this will help you to reduce fear and anxiety, even anger and sadness.

Frequently Asked Questions about Prognosis

- Can I die from this disease?
- Will the disease get worse?
- Can my condition improve?
- Can I still go to school?
- Can I get and keep a job?
- Will I need to be hospitalized?
- Will I need to have surgery?
- Will I need a "bag" outside my body to collect stool?
- What lifestyle changes will I need to make?
- Will I be able to become pregnant?
- Can I take my medication during pregnancy?
- Will my condition flare during pregnancy?
- Will this disease affect the birth of my child?
- Can I travel if I have IBD?

Can I Die from This Disease?

Life Expectancy

Fortunately, death due to IBD is a rare occurrence and, on average, the life expectancy of people with IBD appears to be pretty much the same as people without IBD.

When someone is diagnosed with inflammatory bowel disease, the first thought that may enter the mind is, "Can I die from this disease?" With improvements in the medical and surgical management of IBD, death as a result of IBD or one of its complications is exceedingly rare today, nor is life expectancy shortened.

While some older studies from the 1950s, 1960s, and 1970s suggest that the risk of dying is increased in people with IBD, these studies examined patients who had the disease before many of the modern advances in the medical and surgical care of IBD patients existed, which may have accounted for the slightly higher mortality rate. However, there does appeear to be an increased mortality risk in the first year after diagnosis.

In other instances, surgery may be delayed unnecessarily, leading to more complications and, ultimately, death. Doctors, patients, and their families are sometimes reluctant to consider surgery at the time of diagnosis, even when it may be the most appropriate way of managing the disease if it is very severe. This reluctance may be partly due to the feeling on the part of the doctor that medication should be given a chance to work. Because the patient and the family are not yet familiar with the disease, they may not have come to terms with the need for surgery.

First-Year Risk

Recent studies have suggested that there may still be a slight increased risk of dying in the first year after diagnosis, but after the first year, the risk appears to be no different than in someone without IBD. The reason for this increased risk of dying in the first year after diagnosis is not very clear, but it may be due to the fact that some individuals with IBD will first present with very sudden onset of severe symptoms and severe inflammation, with the result that the correct diagnosis may not be made soon enough to begin proper treatment.

Will the Disease Get Worse?

Predicting the course of the disease in a given individual is very difficult. However, this is something that almost every patient who has been recently diagnosed with IBD wants to know.

Both Crohn's disease and ulcerative colitis are chronic, lifelong disorders that have a tendency to fluctuate in severity over time. The disease seemingly gets better or worse on its own for no apparent reason. It is not uncommon for a person with IBD to be quite well for a period of months or years, only to experience a flare or recurrence of symptoms over a period of days to weeks. Similarly, some people go on for many months or, in some cases, for years with chronic symptoms that do not respond to treatment, only to find that for some reason the symptoms begin to improve on their own.

Risk Profiles

The use of steroid medication for the first flare of disease tends to predict a poorer prognosis. However, this higher risk is probably not entirely due to the medication itself worsening the prognosis; rather, the fact that the doctor chose to use this potent medication indicates that the disease is, in the doctor's overall opinion, relatively severe and requires this medication to treat. In forming this opinion, your doctor typically uses a number of clinical clues based upon her experience that tells her that the patient's disease is more severe and more likely to develop complications or require surgery.

How these clues can help predict the prognosis, for an individual patient, with a high degree of reliability has been the subject of much research. It seems that using individual patient risk profiles, consisting of a combination of factors taken together, may provide the best chance for evaluating prognosis. These risk profiles have traditionally been based upon patient factors and disease factors, such as the age of first diagnosis, location of disease, severity of the first attack, and the appearance of the intestinal lining during colonoscopy.

These work reasonably well, but probably not well enough to help patients and doctors make decisions about disease management in individual patients. More recently, attempts have been made to incorporate blood tests and genetic tests into the risk profiles of patients.

First Attack

There is no question that the severity of the first attack of IBD tends to predict the subsequent course of the disease. Not all of the subsequent flares are necessarily as severe as the first one, but they still cause symptoms, require treatment, and have a significant impact upon a person's life. Patients with first attacks that are less severe tend to have a lower risk of having subsequent flares, but the risk is still present years after the original attack.

Frequency of Flares

When a flare of the disease occurs, there is usually no particular reason that can be identified for it occurring at that particular time in the course of a person's disease. It is natural to try to attribute the flare to various events that may have occurred in someone's life or to various foods that they may have eaten. For example, if you develop a flare of Crohn's disease, you may say that it was because you were eating a lot of junk food or because you are very busy at work, under considerable stress, and not getting enough rest.

Since Crohn's disease and ulcerative colitis are quite variable in their presentation from person to person, it makes sense that the factors causing flares also vary from person to person.

Identifying these factors requires careful observation by patient and doctor to determine what might bring on a flare.

Severity of Disease

Some people will have very mild disease symptoms that don't interfere with their day-to-day activities, whereas others will be almost incapacitated by the severity of the symptoms. It is difficult to predict which category someone will fall into when the disease is first diagnosed.

Similar to the risk of flares, the chance of having more aggressive or severe disease tends to be higher if the first presentation is more severe. Exceptions do occur. Someone may have a severe flare at the first presentation, but once it has settled with treatment, the disease will go into a prolonged period of remission, during which time the person may have very few or no symptoms. This scenario is more common in individuals with ulcerative colitis than with Crohn's disease.

Disease that is very limited — for example, ulcerative colitis affecting only the rectum — may progress and worsen. In this case, the area of inflammation or disease usually remains confined to the rectum and remains stable for many years. However, in approximately 10% to 20% of patients, the inflammation will extend to involve more of the colon, and the patient may become much sicker and more symptomatic when a flare occurs.

Can My Condition Improve?

The severity of Crohn's disease and ulcerative colitis can fluctuate significantly over a period of days, weeks, and months without any apparent reason. Just as a flare can occur in someone who has been quite stable for many months or years, the symptoms of disease can mysteriously improve without any intervention on the part of the doctor and without an obvious cause. Individuals with mild disease may be able to afford to take a chance and wait a little while to see if their situation improves without treatment. That being said, it is unusual for someone with severe disease to improve without any treatment.

Spontaneous Recovery

Mild flares of IBD can sometimes go away without any additional treatment. This phenomenon has been well shown in clinical studies where patients with IBD receive placebo (inactive medication) as a means of comparing a new treatment

---

Increased Flare Risk

It is very difficult to attribute flares to specific life events or to specific foods. Researchers have studied this issue for many years, and no factor — not stress, not diet, not infections — consistently results in increased risk of flares or worsening of the disease.

Disease Extensiveness

The likelihood that the disease will progress or worsen depends, to some degree, on the extent of intestine involved. In general, disease that is more extensive — for example, Crohn's disease that affects long segments of both the small and large intestines — may be more likely to remain active or worsen.

Successful Treatments

Most patients experiencing a flare of ulcerative colitis or Crohn's disease require and request treatment. Patients are often given nutritional advice, with special diets being recommended in specific cases. They may also receive psychological support for managing their symptoms. Although IBD cannot be cured by drug therapy, a number of medications are helpful in reducing inflammation, reducing symptoms, and, in some cases, producing a full remission whereby the patient is free of symptoms. In some cases, surgery may be required, which often has a successful outcome in eliminating or managing symptoms. These various successful treatment strategies are discussed in detail in Part 2 of this book.

Remission

In studies of patients with Crohn's disease and ulcerative colitis, a proportion of the patients who receive no treatment will predictably experience improvement in their symptoms, and in some cases this improvement may be complete (although not necessarily permanent). This spontaneous improvement is more commonly seen in individuals with mild flares or mild symptoms. Simply monitoring a patient with a very mild flare may be a reasonable management approach in some instances.

to no treatment at all. Interestingly, the studies have shown that anywhere from 5% to 30% of patients treated only with placebo will experience improvement. The improvement is not necessarily complete, leading to remission, but it does indicate that the disease can improve without medication.

There have been a number of theories proposed to explain this spontaneous improvement, but no one knows for sure what factors are behind it. Improvements that occur without medication could be due to changes in diet or stress levels, or possibly just a natural day-to-day or week-to-week fluctuation in an individual's immune response. Researchers are working to determine why disease flares occur and how spontaneous improvements occur. This information may help to develop new ways of preventing disease flares and treating IBD.

Can I Still Go to School?

Because school-age children and young adults are the ones who are often diagnosed with Crohn's disease or ulcerative colitis, these diseases can potentially interfere with getting an education.

Let your teachers know that you have IBD and explain the symptoms so they understand that you may be absent from school because of flares and doctor appointments. Teachers can accommodate students who may need to be excused during class or during an exam to go to the bathroom. If you need to be away from school for a prolonged period of time, for hospitalization or surgery, you may be able to arrange for assignments to be brought to you by friends or classmates. Some hospitals provide Internet access for patients who want to keep up on their studies. Some schools use the Internet extensively to post assignments and to provide a forum for feedback from teachers.

However, when you are sick and in hospital, you may not feel up to working or reading. Your ability to concentrate may be reduced. If you happen to be away from school for many weeks at a time and have not been able to keep up with work from home or hospital, you may require additional help from the teachers or tutors in order to catch up. In post-secondary education, because of the intensive nature of the workload and the relatively short semesters, catching up may not always be possible. In some instances, you may need to take a leave or drop some courses and make them up the following term. You can ask your doctor to write a supporting letter. Although it may take you longer to complete your degree or diploma requirements, you will be less stressed and get more rest.

A minority of students have symptoms that are severe enough or persistent enough to cause them to have to change their educational objectives. It is the unpredictability of the disease that causes IBD patients to change their school plans. Frequent disease flares in people with more severe disease can require relatively long absences from school, which can, in turn, have a negative effect on grades.

Discrimination

You may fear that prospective employers will disqualify you for a job once they learn about your condition. However, you are not required to disclose illnesses or disabilities to a prospective employer, nor can the employer discriminate against someone based upon a disability. In the province of Ontario, for example, the Ontario Human Rights Code prohibits discrimination in employment based upon disability. In the United States, the federal disability laws forbid most employers from asking about the medical conditions of an applicant, although the United States Supreme Court has ruled that an employer can refuse to hire someone who has a chronic condition that may be made worse by the job. Precise laws and rulings vary from jurisdiction to jurisdiction, so it is best to check with human resources specialists, career or hiring coaches, or lawyers when deciding on whether to disclose your condition to a prospective employer.

Can I Get and Keep a Job?

There are many IBD sufferers who have successfully completed their education and gone on to a variety of successful careers as teachers, executives, entrepreneurs, lawyers, professors, engineers, police officers, farmers, doctors, nurses, authors, artists, and professional athletes. IBD does not necessarily mean that you will be limited in your choice of careers or that you cannot excel at your job.

Disclosure

Employers may feel deceived if the condition is not disclosed to them during the interview process and the applicant then becomes ill or incapacitated shortly after hiring. You can take this opportunity to educate your employers about your condition, though you don't need to give the details of all of your symptoms. In the end, you have to decide for yourself how much to disclose to the employer during the job interview process.

Keep in mind the perspective of your employers. They may not know much about the condition and may wonder if it will affect your work performance, if the disease is likely to progress, if the job will impact upon your condition, and if any modification in schedule or duties is required. Be prepared to answer these questions honestly. In addition to developing a more trusting relationship with the employer, disclosure may result in a more flexible work schedule or work conditions. Alternatively, you can make it clear that you don't expect any special treatment.

Disability

Although the majority of IBD sufferers are able to get and keep good jobs, there is a small proportion who have flares so frequently, or who have some degree of symptoms almost continuously, that they are not able to work. Eventually, they may need to go on short-term or long-term disability. Sometimes they are able to resume working on a limited basis if the disease can be controlled through medical or surgical management. Some people with severe symptoms gravitate to jobs where the employer is more sympathetic to their special needs or to jobs where there may be more flexibility in work hours. Many large companies have disability counselors who help people make the transition back into the workplace on a gradual basis by finding appropriate positions and work schedules that fit with their chronic symptoms.

Fortunately, most people with IBD are able to continue working in their usual job. Surveys have shown that more than 80% are ultimately able to carry on with their usual activities.

More Understanding

Even if disclosure is not required by law, some people with chronic medical conditions prefer to disclose their condition to the employer during the interview process. If you disclose your illness to your employers, you may find that they are more understanding when you do have to take the occasional day or two off work because of your condition.

There does appear to be an increase in time missed from school or work in the first year or two after the first diagnosis of IBD, but after that, the number of days missed from work is, on average, not much different from those people who do not have IBD. However, it may take several years after diagnosis for someone to get back on track.

Success Stories

Most IBD sufferers are able to lead happy and productive lives, pursuing a career that appeals to them and fits with their abilities. These people are usually able to succeed because they see their disease as just another challenge to overcome in achieving their career goals, the same way that they need to pass a school exam, develop an innovative ad campaign, or perfect a new surgical technique. Fortunately, it is only the very rare individual who is not able to pursue their chosen career path solely because of their IBD.

Will I Need to Be Hospitalized?

In the past, hospitalization for IBD patients was very common, especially at the time of first diagnosis. In recent years, disease flares have been managed on an outpatient basis, with hospitalization reserved primarily for very severe disease flares, for complications of the disease, and for surgery. Many physicians now realize that, in most cases, hospitalization is not needed to provide effective medical therapy or to properly monitor a patient's response to therapy.

However, outpatient treatment requires more time and effort on the part of the physician and other members of the health-care team. Health-care professionals now spend more time educating patients and their families about what to expect from the therapy and what to look for in the way of side effects or potential complications. This requires close communication between the treatment team — the physician or nurse clinician — and the patient and family.

Managing Unpredictability

The unpredictability of IBD can make it very difficult for some people to deal with Crohn's disease or ulcerative colitis. Planning your day-to-day activities, let alone your life, when the possibility of a flare or worsening of the disease hangs over your head is not easy. You will need to develop ways of becoming more flexible to cope with this unpredictability.

Will I Need to Have Surgery?

On average, 20% to 34% of ulcerative colitis patients and 70% to 80% of Crohn's disease patients will require surgery at some point in the course of their disease.

The likelihood of requiring surgery depends, to a large extent, on how well the disease responds to non-surgical treatments, such as nutritional support or medications. Surgery also depends on the severity, extent, and location of the disease. Patients and families should keep in mind that hospitalization and surgery are not the same as admitting defeat, and that many IBD sufferers go on to lead very fulfilling lives with many years free from recurrent disease following surgery.

In ulcerative colitis, surgery is said to "cure" the disease, although it does leave the individual with a different internal and, occasionally, external anatomy. There are also some risks of complications of surgery. Unfortunately, in individuals with Crohn's disease, many operations carry a risk of possible recurrence of the disease in areas of the intestine that were not affected before surgery.

Will I Need a "Bag" Outside My Body to Collect Stool?

Occasionally, the surgeon must bring part of the intestine out to the skin so that the waste material (stool) collects in a bag, a procedure known as a stoma. Two main types of stomas are performed in IBD patients: an ileostomy, which involves bringing the last part of the small intestine out to the skin; and a colostomy, which involves bringing the large intestine out to the skin. These two types of stomas are somewhat different in their appearance and function.

Many patients fear the possibility of surgery because they believe that this means that they will be left with a stoma for the rest of their lives. Fortunately, this situation is the exception rather than the rule. The stoma can be reversed by another operation several months after the first. Even when a permanent stoma is required, a person can lead a normal life with good health and an active lifestyle. This requires some adjustment and support, but it can almost always be achieved.

What Lifestyle Changes Will I Need to Make?

Stress, fatigue, colds, flu, medications, smoking, alcohol, and other lifestyle factors appear to have an impact upon Crohn's disease and ulcerative colitis. Although researchers have tried

Main Lifestyle Factors

Certain lifestyle factors will increase the likelihood that a flare of IBD will occur. The main factors are stress and use of non-steroidal anti-inflammatory drugs. There is more to a disease flare or worsening than a single factor. It is likely that several factors, many of which we probably don't fully understand, work together to increase the likelihood of a flare.

to prove the connection between these factors and disease severity, it is very difficult to prove scientifically that these associations exist. How does one measure stress or fatigue? How can you be certain that the cold you had 2 weeks ago is causing your disease to flare up now? Are two or three doses of an anti-inflammatory medication taken for a headache enough to cause increased symptoms?

There is really nothing that will guarantee that a flare will occur in a given individual. You may find that you experienced a flare during final exams in your first year of university — a time of great stress for most students — but the following year, you sailed through an equally difficult exam schedule without a disease flare.

Stress and Fatigue

Stress is often associated with disturbed sleep patterns and fatigue. Fatigue can affect immune system functioning and, possibly, IBD flares. Fatigue is a symptom of IBD that can be very difficult to treat, but it is generally considered good advice to obtain sufficient sleep and rest, particularly if you feel a flare coming on.

If you are able to get a good night's sleep but still wake feeling unrested, or if you become quickly tired during the day and have to lie down, it may be that your disease is active and causing you to feel fatigue. In some cases, even minimal inflammation of the intestine — not enough to cause any other symptoms — may produce very profound fatigue. In other instances, a vitamin or mineral deficiency, such as iron, folic acid, or vitamin B_{12} deficiency, can lead to fatigue. In those instances, appropriate supplementation can correct the symptom.

Smoking

Smoking has many related health risks. In addition to its deleterious effects on the lungs and heart, smoking may also be detrimental to Crohn's disease. Smoking tends to increase the risk of Crohn's disease first developing, and once someone has Crohn's disease, it makes the disease more aggressive. Disease seems to come back more quickly and aggressively after surgery in smokers. If you are a smoker and have Crohn's disease, you can do yourself a big favor and quit. Get all of the help you can — support from family and friends (even if they are smokers and have to quit too) and from your doctor or health-care provider for referral to smoking cessation programs or prescriptions for drugs that can help you kick the habit.

Impaired Sleep

If you are not sleeping well, it may be because of your disease symptoms, such as frequent diarrhea at night, but if you are not sleeping well despite the absence of symptoms, you should discuss this with your doctor. Impaired sleep can be a sign of anxiety or depression and proper treatment can improve your sleep patterns.

However, smoking actually appears to be protective against developing ulcerative colitis. For patients with ulcerative colitis who are former smokers, the period soon after smoking cessation seems to be a time of particularly increased risk of developing this disease. In the occasional ulcerative colitis patient who happens to be a smoker, the disease may become more active after smoking cessation. This observation has even led some researchers to use nicotine, in the form of skin patches, as a treatment for ulcerative colitis.

Despite the strong association between cigarette smoking and protection against ulcerative colitis, this approach to treatment has not been proven to be consistently effective. If you are a non-smoker and you develop ulcerative colitis, don't start smoking, because other health risks outweigh any possible benefit that you might get from smoking.

Will I Be Able to Become Pregnant?

If your condition is under good control, you should expect to have as much chance of getting pregnant as a woman who does not have IBD. However, when the disease is active, it can get in the way of pregnancy.

If you are quite sick with a disease flare, you probably don't feel like becoming pregnant — and you may not be able to. Your symptoms and any resulting weight loss can interrupt your normal menstrual cycle, so that your ovaries may not be releasing an egg every month. If there are no eggs being released, there can be no pregnancy. Fortunately, when you recover from a flare of IBD, the menstrual cycle tends to become more regular again, the ovulation (release of eggs) resumes, and pregnancy is possible.

Surgery for IBD or complications of IBD, particularly abscesses from Crohn's disease, can also lead to increased rates of infertility, probably due to scarring around the fallopian tubes, which carry the egg from the ovary to the uterus. Complications of surgery, such as a leak or an abscess, increase the rate of fertility problems even further.

Although disease flares tend to make becoming pregnant more difficult, it is not a guarantee that you will not become pregnant. If you are sexually active during a disease flare and do not want to be pregnant, you should use appropriate birth control methods.

> ### Caution Before Surgery
>
> Before any surgery for IBD or its complications, be sure to inform your surgeon about your plans for having children and ask what procedure would best meet your needs.

Can I Take My Medication during Pregnancy?

Most medications that are used for the treatment of IBD can be used during pregnancy if they are truly needed to bring the disease under control or to maintain remission in someone who has had a very rocky course. However, do not take methotrexate. There is also some concern about the use of ciprofloxacin and its effect on cartilage development in the fetus. By all means, the 5-ASA containing medications and steroids, such as prednisone, can be used during pregnancy and appear to be exceedingly safe with respect to their effects on the fetus and the mother.

During your pregnancy, you should be followed closely by a gastroenterologist or other expert in IBD, as well as an obstetrician. Some health centers have high-risk obstetrics units for pregnant women with chronic underlying medical conditions, such as Crohn's disease or ulcerative colitis.

Will My Condition Flare during Pregnancy?

If the disease is active when you become pregnant, there is a high likelihood that it will remain active throughout the pregnancy. However, there is a significant proportion of women who say that they "never felt as well" as they did when they were pregnant. Many of them say that they wish they could figure out how to be pregnant all of the time so that their IBD remains under control. If the disease is in remission at the beginning of the pregnancy, but becomes active later on during pregnancy, it can be treated as needed with most medications normally used in non-pregnant women, with the exception of methotrexate.

Will this Disease Affect the Birth of My Child?

Women with IBD are usually able to carry the baby to term, although there does seem to be a slightly higher rate of early or premature delivery in IBD patients, particularly if the disease is active during pregnancy. In addition, there is also a tendency to have babies that are slightly small for their gestational age.

Episiotomies are perfectly fine if they avoid an uncontrolled tear into the anal sphincter or rectum. The only time when a Caesarian section might be considered solely because of the IBD and not for obstetrical reasons is in a woman with Crohn's disease who has complicated perianal disease with a lot of inflammation and possible infection around the anus and the vagina. In that particular situation, a Caesarian section is probably the safest way to go.

If you have IBD, you can expect to have as much chance as any other woman of having a vaginal delivery. However, it is important for the delivering obstetrician to be aware that you have IBD and to avoid an uncontrolled tear.

Can I Travel If I Have IBD?

Traveling for business or pleasure and visiting with friends and family members far from home can often be stressful for IBD sufferers. When you are feeling well and your IBD is well controlled, you shouldn't feel hindered in your travel. If the disease is active or has been quite unpredictable, you might be best to delay your travel plans if at all possible until things are more stable. There is nothing worse than having to spend most of your time on vacation inside a hotel room because you are experiencing symptoms of IBD.

Not only do IBD symptoms make you feel bad, but you will probably feel doubly bad because you are missing out on fun and good times. That is not to say you should not travel out of fear that a flare might occur while you are away; instead, you should try to choose the best time to travel based upon how you are feeling and how your disease has behaved in the past. If you are not sure, you can talk to your doctor about your travel plans.

Many people with IBD find that travel, whether due to the change in routine or the change in diet, can cause changes in the way their gastrointestinal tract functions. Diarrhea, cramping, increased gas, and abdominal distension can all occur. Traveling can be quite tiring, especially if it involves long periods in a car, bus, train, or airplane or travel across many time zones. In most cases, the symptoms experienced do not necessarily represent a flare of the disease, but are something that can be experienced by anyone, whether or not they have IBD.

> **Traveling Precautions**
>
> Speak with your doctor about what precautions you might take against traveler's diarrhea. Some doctors will provide a prescription for a supply of antibiotics to be taken if you develop diarrhea, rectal bleeding, and fever. However, the best treatment is prevention by being careful.

Traveler's Diarrhea

When you travel, you often eat food that you have not prepared yourself and you may not be sure where the food originated. As a result, there may be a chance that you can pick up "traveler's diarrhea." This is a catch-all term for a variety of different infections caused by viruses and bacteria that may be transmitted by eating contaminated food or drinking contaminated water.

There are certain countries or locations that are well known as being places where people can pick up traveler's diarrhea if they are not careful about what they eat and drink. Most often these are tropical destinations. Although some of the resort areas or hotels have reasonably safe food and water supplies, you should still be careful about drinking unbottled water or drinks with ice or eating salads, unpeeled fruits, and vegetables. In general, anything that is uncooked and that might have been washed with contaminated water is best to avoid. Definitely avoid eating food from street vendors.

Travel Rx

Certain precautions and preparations need to be undertaken when you are traveling with IBD. These will vary from individual to individual, depending on the severity of the disease, its symptoms and complications, the medications being taken, and the presence of a stoma bag.

- If you are not traveling alone, try to choose traveling companions who understand your disease and the symptoms you might experience. Be honest with them. For example, you can tell them, "I have to make sure that I have a bathroom break at least every 2 hours." The travel itinerary can be planned accordingly.

- If you are traveling by plane, try to plan your bathroom visits away from times when the bathroom is busiest — usually after meals or first thing in the morning on overnight flights. Try to use the bathroom just before getting on a plane, train, or bus or before getting into a lineup at the check-in counter, security, or customs. Some people find it helpful to take an antidiarrheal medication, such as Imodium or Lomotil, just before boarding or before going on a long car trip. This can reduce the amount of diarrhea and urgency, providing some feeling of security. However, this is not safe for all people with IBD or in all situations. Be sure to check with your doctor before trying this approach.

- If loss of bowel control is a possibility or something that you worry about, make sure that you have a change of clothes and have some premoistened disposable towelettes in your carry-on luggage.

- Take time to rest and to eat regular meals. Ideally, these meals should be nutritious, but this isn't always possible on the road. When on an airplane, it is sometimes best to eat lightly and avoid foods and drinks containing caffeine — coffee, chocolates, and cola drinks — which can increase diarrhea.

- Make sure that you maintain an adequate fluid intake (preferably water), especially if you are feeling dehydrated and thirsty. As a general rule, approximately 6 to 8 glasses (1.5 to 2 L) a day should be adequate.

- If you are traveling by plane or across international borders and you are taking medications with you, take the medications in the original bottle or box that you obtained from the pharmacy, along with the pharmacy label indicating your name, the drug's name, and the physician's name. If you are traveling to another country, write down the generic name of the medications because the brand names are frequently different in different countries.

- If you are traveling with medication that requires needles or syringes, ask for a letter from your physician that describes your diagnosis and indicates your need for medication given by injection. This is absolutely necessary if you are planning on taking the medication and supplies with you as a carry-on onto an airplane. This also pertains to supplies for an ostomy.

- Ensure that your medications are not exposed to extreme temperatures (hot or cold) for prolonged periods. The same goes for stoma supplies. If you are traveling by car, don't leave the medication or supplies in the trunk or in the back seat of the car on a hot summer day or a frigid winter day. If you have medication that requires cold storage, consider the use of an insulated carrying bag with freezer packs.

- Take more medication and supplies with you than you think you will need. Some people like to pack some in their checked luggage and keep some in their carry-on luggage.

What Causes IBD?

Although the potential impact of Crohn's disease and ulcerative colitis on your life is the most pressing concern at the time of diagnosis, you will probably also want to know how you could have possibly developed this illness. The factors that may contribute to the development of IBD and how researchers are looking for the causes of IBD are discussed in the next chapter.

CHAPTER 4

How Did I Get This Disease?

CASE STUDY Allison

Allison is a 27-year-old woman who works as a salesperson at a retail store. She is engaged to be married. She finds this time in her life to be very exciting but also very stressful.

Her 25-year-old brother has had Crohn's disease since he was 20. Allison has generally been quite healthy, but she smokes half a pack of cigarettes a day. She has had progressive abdominal cramps, rectal bleeding, and diarrhea for the past 2 months. She recently went to a hospital emergency department with a painful swelling near the anus. The surgeon who examined her drained what turned out to be an abscess.

Because of her history, the surgeon referred her to a gastroenterologist, who carried out a number of tests, including a colonoscopy, and found that she had Crohn's disease of both her small and large intestines. He informed her of the diagnosis and prescribed several medications.

After the shock of the new diagnosis wore off, Allison had a number of questions, but by then she had been discharged from hospital and her next appointment with the specialist was not for another 4 weeks. She notices that two of the medications she has been prescribed are antibiotics, but she has heard from her brother that Crohn's disease is not due to an infection. However, a close friend has told her that she read that Crohn's disease is caused by an unusual type of tuberculosis and can be cured by taking antibiotics against tuberculosis.

Allison wonders what has actually caused her to develop Crohn's disease. Is it an infection? Could stress have played a role? Because her brother also has Crohn's disease, could it be genetic? Could it be something in the food that they ate when they were children? Could it be due to the food she eats now? Could it be related somehow to the fact that she smokes cigarettes? The list of possible causes seemed endless.

Research Models

There are many methods by which researchers work to uncover the causes of IBD and discover why it occurs in certain individuals and not in others:

- Experiments done in test tubes using single cells or cells grown in a culture
- Experiments done in animals that develop IBD either spontaneously or through some type of experimental manipulation
- Experiments done on genetic samples taken from humans
- Experiments done on bacteria present in the intestines of IBD patients
- Experiments testing different treatment approaches in humans
- Research studies looking at factors that may predict who does and who doesn't get IBD
- Studies examining environmental factors, such as geographic location, diet, intestinal bacteria, and chemical exposures, to name a few, that might promote or protect against the development of IBD

Several theories about the cause of IBD and the intestinal inflammation process have emerged since Crohn's disease and ulcerative colitis were first described:

- IBD is an infection
- IBD is an inherited or acquired immune deficiency
- IBD is an overactive immune system acting against itself (autoimmunity)
- IBD is a reaction to some recognized or unrecognized factor in the environment
- IBD is a genetic disorder

Although researchers often believe that their own method of research will uncover the causes of IBD and, ultimately, the cure, the various methods really complement one another. It is highly likely that IBD will be found to be due to multiple factors — both those that we inherit from our parents (genetic factors) and those that we are exposed to in the food we eat, the infections we acquire, and the chemicals and toxins we may be exposed to (environmental factors).

Causal Factors

When patients are told that they have inflammatory bowel disease, the first question they will likely ask is, "What is this disease?" The next question that is foremost in most people's minds concerns their pressing symptoms and their prognosis. Once the diagnosis of IBD is confirmed and the prognosis understood, they begin to question, "How did I get this disease?" Logically, understanding the causes of the disease should lead to developing a "cure." However, the causes of inflammatory bowel disease have not been determined conclusively. There appear to be a number of causal factors — and a number of corresponding treatments.

Although there have been major advances in our understanding of what happens when the bowel becomes inflamed in inflammatory bowel disease, we still do not know exactly what causes this condition. We also do not know what triggers the process of intestinal inflammation or why one person may develop it whereas a neighbor, brother, sister, or child may not. This apparent lack of research progress can be frustrating for patients and their families.

However, there has been no lack of effort to crack the mysteries of Crohn's disease and ulcerative colitis. From these research studies, we have come to recognize that there may not be a single cause that explains every manifestation of inflammatory bowel disease in every individual; instead, the disease may have many causes that interact to produce IBD in a previously healthy individual.

Possible Infectious Causes

There are many similarities between the way IBD presents in the intestines and a number of specific infections caused by bacteria, viruses, and parasites. Well-recognized intestinal infections, caused by specific bacteria (such as salmonella, campylobacter, yersinia, several strains of E. coli), by specific viruses (such as Norwalk virus and rotavirus), and by parasites (such as *Entamoeba histolytica* and giardia), often produce intestinal inflammation and damage, along with the associated symptoms of abdominal pain, diarrhea, and rectal bleeding, but they do not usually last more than several days before they are cleared by the body's immune system. These microbes (bacteria, viruses, and parasites) typically do not produce chronic or long-lasting intestinal inflammation and have not been found in the intestines or stools of patients with IBD. They usually do not recur once the microbe is cleared by the immune system, unless a person is exposed again to the microbe in question.

Bacteria

Although it appears unlikely that a disease-causing (pathogenic) bacterium is the cause of IBD, the thousands of billions of bacteria from the hundreds of bacteria species normally present in the intestine may somehow contribute to the inflammatory process. No single bacterial species or strain is solely responsible for the inflammatory effect; it requires a particular combination of strains to induce inflammation in someone who is genetically susceptible.

Clostridium difficile

One particular bacterial infection, called *Clostridium difficile*, is found in the stool of IBD patients from time to time, particularly during a flare of the disease. However, *Clostridium difficile* is not known to cause IBD; rather, IBD likely provides suitable conditions for the growth of this bacterial species.

L-Forms

Other bacteria that do not cause infection may contribute to the cause of IBD. Researchers have experimented with bacteria that were missing their cell wall as a possible cause. It was thought that these bacteria, called L-forms, could produce chronic infection that is indistinguishable from IBD. Subsequent studies have shown that these bacterial forms are not involved in IBD.

Mycobacteria

Another species of mycobacterium, called *Mycobacterium paratuberculosis*, produces Johne's disease in cattle. Johne's disease looks somewhat like Crohn's disease in humans. Prevalent in dairy herds and excreted in milk from infected cows, this bacterium is not completely killed by the pasteurization of milk and is, therefore, potentially present in the milk supply. Some experts have suggested that *Mycobacterium paratuberculosis* may be able to infect humans and that this chronic infection may be the cause of Crohn's disease, in at least some patients.

In some studies, researchers have been able to detect antibodies against specific segments of mycobacterial proteins in the blood of human Crohn's disease patients, and in other studies, they have been able to detect genetic sequences specific to mycobacteria in inflamed intestinal tissues of Crohn's disease patients.

Some investigators have apparently had success in treating Crohn's disease using regimens consisting of multiple antibiotics that are active against *Mycobacterium paratuberculosis*. However, the number of patients treated has been relatively small, and most researchers have not been able to reproduce the findings of mycobacteria in the intestinal tissues or the response to therapy against mycobacteria.

Tuberculosis

Some researchers have suggested that the bacteria causing tuberculosis in humans might be the cause of Crohn's disease. *Mycobacterium tuberculosis* can infect the intestines, and the appearance of Crohn's disease has some similarities to intestinal tuberculosis. However, careful study of intestinal tissues from Crohn's disease patients has not shown tuberculosis infection to be a cause.

Viruses

Microbes other than bacteria can cause intestinal inflammation and have, therefore, also been considered as possible causes of IBD. Viruses, in particular, may be very difficult to detect in the intestinal lining or in stool samples, and it has been speculated that a virus that has eluded detection may be the cause of IBD.

Paramyxoviruses (Measles)

Paramyxoviruses, of which the measles virus is the best known, has received considerable attention. By using blood testing to detect antibodies directed against paramyxovirus or by using very powerful electron microscopy on biopsy and surgical resection specimens, some investigators have found what they believe to be evidence of a paramyxovirus infection in Crohn's disease patients. However, recent studies using very sensitive genetic probes for paramyxovirus have not been able to detect this evidence of measles virus.

Subsequently, the proponents of the "measles theory" have suggested that it is not necessarily an actual infection by measles virus that produces Crohn's disease, but rather the late effects of early childhood infection or exposure of one's mother to measles virus during pregnancy. They have also suggested that Crohn's disease may be a result of childhood immunization against measles using the live measles vaccine, in which the virus is still alive but cannot produce the usual measles infection. There is some indirect evidence supporting this theory, but it consists mainly of the apparent increase in the incidence of Crohn's disease following the institution of universal measles vaccination programs in developed countries in the 1960s.

Possible Environmental Causes

There are differences in the prevalence of Crohn's disease and ulcerative colitis between countries, as well as between ethnic groups within a given country. These differences have led scientists to suggest that, in addition to infections, other environmental factors, such as toxins, diet, smoking, medication use, and even geography, may have a significant influence on the development of IBD.

Twin Studies

We know that environmental factors influence IBD from studies of twins. When one identical twin has Crohn's disease or ulcerative colitis, the other twin, who is genetically identical, will not necessarily develop IBD. To produce the disease, some environmental influence or exposure must interact with the genetic background that makes a person susceptible to developing IBD. Presumably, one twin has been exposed to disease-causing environmental factors, while the other has not been exposed to those factors or has not been exposed for long enough or exposed at the right time in the course of growth and development.

Population Studies

Researchers have tried to determine what some of these environmental factors might be in a number of ways. Often, they will take a group of IBD patients and find out about various possible risk factors that they might have been exposed to and compare them to a group of similar individuals who do not have IBD. Researchers will also examine where people with IBD were born and where they grew up while looking for clues to possible environmental exposures.

Through these studies, it has been discovered that the incidence of IBD is highest in developed North American and Northern European countries and lower in less developed or more southerly countries. This has raised the theory that something we are exposed to in developed countries contributes to the development of IBD. An interesting observation is the change in the pattern of IBD in other areas of the world. In Japan, for example, Crohn's disease was almost unheard of in 1950, but the incidence of the disease has risen steadily since then. This increase has been explained by some experts as the result of a change in the Japanese diet. During the time that Crohn's disease has increased in Japan, the diet has become increasingly Westernized, with less traditional rice and fish and more red meat being eaten. However, the change in diet and the increase in incidence do not prove cause and effect, since many other aspects of life in Japan changed between 1950 and the present time.

Diet

Dietary factors are obvious potential risk factors, given that Crohn's disease and ulcerative colitis are intestinal disorders. Food comes into direct contact with the intestinal lining. Although no specific food or food category has been consistently found to be a potential triggering factor in IBD, some studies have found that diets that are high in red meat or refined sugars may increase the risk of developing IBD.

Environmental Triggers

IBD patients may experience spontaneous improvements and relapses. However, we do not know what induces or triggers a change in the degree of inflammation in the intestines. Despite extensive research, we cannot say for certain what environmental factors may trigger the disease initially or may result in exacerbations once the disease is established.

Breast-feeding Protection

Children who have been breast-fed may be at lower risk of subsequently developing IBD than children who have been formula-fed. If true, this would mean that there is something potentially harmful in infant formula or, more likely, something protective in breast milk.

Altering dietary intake may result in improvement in intestinal inflammation and symptoms of disease. This is not to say that dietary factors cause IBD, but once IBD is established, modification of the diet may, in some instances, improve the disease activity and symptoms.

There may be some factor in the diet that worsens or propagates the inflammatory reaction in the intestines of IBD patients. It is not clear what this factor or factors might be. Attempts at carrying out exclusion or elimination diets, in which specific foods are removed from and then added back into the diet one at a time, have not identified a specific food trigger in the majority of patients.

Hygiene

In recent years, there has been interest in the so-called hygiene hypothesis to explain a number of chronic inflammatory or autoimmune diseases, such as asthma. As a result of living in an increasingly clean and hygienic society, we are not exposed to many of the infections that we once were. This is particularly true in the early childhood years. As a result, a person's immune system may become overactive because it is not accustomed to dealing with bacteria, viruses, and parasites. This leads to increased immune or inflammatory responses to proteins, bacteria, and viruses that would not have been considered "foreign" or would not have produced such a vigorous and damaging response in the past.

Environmental Exposures

Since the appearance of IBD seems to have coincided with the advent of modern industrialized society, other aspects of our modern society are being explored as important environmental factors that have, in some way, contributed to the rise in IBD. Prominent among these are airborne environmental pollutants caused by internal combustion vehicles and by industry. Studies investigating the numerous possible environmental exposures are still at a relatively early stage, but there are certain environmental pollutants or toxins that theoretically may have an impact upon the immune system.

Smoking

The relationship between cigarette smoking and IBD has long been known. Patients with ulcerative colitis are more likely to be non-smokers or former smokers, and patients with Crohn's disease are more likely to be smokers. How cigarette smoking interacts with other factors to either increase or decrease the risk of disease is entirely unknown.

Medications

Some medications are known to cause irritation and even damage to the lining of the intestinal tract. Aspirin and non-steroidal anti-inflammatory drugs (for example, ibuprofen, naproxen, diclofenac, and sulindac) are well known to cause ulcers in the stomach and duodenum. These drugs can also have damaging effects on the lining of the intestinal tract in the last part of the small intestine (ileum) and the large intestine, the areas most commonly affected in IBD.

No Drug Cause

Despite the potential for tissue damage and the risk of a flare when using aspirin and non-steroidal anti-inflammatory drugs, these drugs have not been shown to cause Crohn's disease or ulcerative colitis.

Possible Inherited (Genetic) Factors

Crohn's disease and ulcerative colitis have a tendency to run in families. This inherited susceptibility to the disease is carried within the genetic code. The genetic code is present, at some point in development, in every cell of the human body and is passed down from parent to child. Recent research has shown that there are maybe 100 inherited susceptibility factors (genes) that, when altered, can increase a person's chances of developing Crohn's disease and 50 associated with ulcerative colitis. Some of these genes appear to be specific to Crohn's disease risk, some appear to be specific to ulcerative colitis, and some appear to be shared by the two disorders.

Twin Studies

In studies of twins, in which at least one twin has IBD, it has been found that if one twin has Crohn's disease, the likelihood that the other twin also has Crohn's disease is much higher if the twins are genetically identical than if the twins are not genetically identical (fraternal twins). Since both identical twins and fraternal twins tend to share the same non-inherited factors, such as diet and environmental exposures, the higher risk in identical twins means that a genetic, or inherited, factor must be playing an important role in causing disease susceptibility.

Gene Basics

Genes contain the code that determines most of the physical characteristics of a person, animal, or plant. Not only do genes determine a person's height, hair and eye color, and blood type, they also determine a person's susceptibility to developing a wide range of diseases and disorders.

- Genes are made up of a molecule called deoxyribonucleic acid (DNA). There are tens of thousands of genes in every human being, each one coded for one of tens of thousands of corresponding proteins that are produced by the cells and tissues of a person. Through these protein products, the genes are able to determine a person's physical characteristics or disease susceptibility.

- Each gene is made up of a series of molecule fragments, called bases. The sequence of these bases — there are four bases in total, represented by the letters A, T, C, and G — tells the body how to make the protein in question. If one or more of these letters are missing or out of order, or if one or more extra letters are present in the wrong place (also known as mutations), the protein that is produced may be defective or it may not be produced at all.

- Each person has two copies of each gene — one inherited from the mother and one inherited from the father. Some diseases require just one of the two copies to be abnormal in order to produce disease, whereas other diseases require both copies to be abnormal. In some diseases, the risk is increased only slightly with one abnormal copy and increased to a much greater extent when two abnormal copies are present.

Genetic Risk

Approximately 10% to 20% of individuals with IBD have another affected family member. If someone within a family has Crohn's disease or ulcerative colitis, the chance of an unaffected member of the family developing IBD is as high as 10%, depending on the nature of the relationship and whether the individual has Crohn's disease or ulcerative colitis. In general, Crohn's disease appears to have a greater tendency to run in families.

Human Genome

Researchers have identified approximately 100 genes that appear to influence the likelihood of developing Crohn's disease or ulcerative colitis. Some seem to be specific to Crohn's disease, some appear to be more specific to ulcerative colitis, and a few appear to be associated with both diseases.

- One of the major breakthroughs in the field of IBD genetics has been the discovery that a gene called CARD15 (also referred to as NOD-2) can result in susceptibility to developing Crohn's disease. When one of the two copies of the CARD15 gene is mutated, thereby resulting in an abnormal or absent protein product, the risk of developing Crohn's disease is approximately doubled or tripled. If both copies of the CARD15 gene are abnormal, the risk of developing Crohn's disease is as much as 30 times greater than if both copies of the gene are normal.

- There are three common abnormalities of the CARD15 gene, any one of which can result in the increased risk. Mutations in the CARD15 gene may be responsible for as much as 20% of Crohn's disease in populations of European background. When the CARD15 gene is abnormal, various cells in the body, in particular immune reactive cells, can produce either an abnormal version of the CARD15 protein or they don't produce the CARD15 protein at all.

- The CARD15 gene product appears to be involved in the part of a person's immune response that is important in fighting off certain bacterial infections or responding to the by-products of certain bacteria. This may mean that CARD15 gene mutations can cause a disruption of this part of the immune response to bacteria. This may lead to an abnormal interaction between the human host and the bacteria in the intestines. This abnormal interaction may then lead to uncontrolled intestinal inflammation and IBD.

- Some of the other genes that have been possibly linked to the development of IBD may be involved in maintaining the barrier function of the intestinal lining. When the barrier function of the intestine is defective, it may be possible for large molecules, such as proteins and intestinal bacteria, to cross into the bowel wall. These proteins and bacteria, which are considered to be "foreign" by the person's immune system, can then cause an inflammatory reaction. This inflammatory reaction is normally intended to eliminate the foreign protein or bacteria, but in IBD, the reaction is not properly controlled or regulated.

- Other genes associated with IBD are, like the NOD-2/CARD15 gene, responsible for the response to bacteria. Another group of genes is responsible for the process of cellular "housekeeping," which results in elimination of debris within cells and also causes old or damaged cells to undergo elimination. Yet another group of genes associated with IBD are responsible for various aspects of the body's immune response.

Q What is the risk to a brother or sister of a person with IBD?

A When a person has Crohn's disease, siblings have an approximately 1 in 12 chance of developing inflammatory bowel disease, either Crohn's disease or ulcerative colitis, in their lifetime. The risk of developing Crohn's disease is probably 5 times that of ulcerative colitis. When a person has ulcerative colitis, siblings have approximately a 1 in 20 chance of developing IBD in their lifetime. In that instance, the risk of ulcerative colitis is likely twice the risk of Crohn's disease.

Q What is the risk to a child of a mother or father with IBD?

A When a father or mother has Crohn's disease, their children have approximately a 1 in 15 chance of developing IBD in their lifetime. The risk is 3 to 5 times higher when the parent has Crohn's disease rather than ulcerative colitis. When a parent has ulcerative colitis, the children have approximately a 1 in 25 chance of developing IBD in their lifetime. When the parent has ulcerative colitis, the type of IBD that a child may develop is more likely to be ulcerative colitis than it is to be Crohn's disease. In that instance, ulcerative colitis is approximately twice as likely as Crohn's disease.

It does not seem to matter whether it is the father or mother who has IBD when discussing the risk to the child. The disease can be passed down from either parent. When both parents have IBD, which is unusual, the children have a much higher risk of developing IBD than would be the case if only one parent has IBD. While it is difficult to provide an exact estimate of what this risk to a child of two affected parents would be, it is probably more than 1 chance in 10 and possibly as much as 1 chance in 3.

Q **What is the risk to a parent of a person with IBD?**

A Although the risk to a parent is very low if a child has IBD, it is still higher than it would be if the mother or father didn't have any family history of IBD. In most instances where a child and parent both have IBD, the parent has usually developed the disease first, and the child has developed the disease some time after it has developed in the parent. This is usually many years later.

Q **I have IBD… what can I do to prevent my child from developing IBD in the future?**

A Although a family history of IBD involving a parent or a sibling is the strongest known risk factor for developing the disease, there really is not much that can be done to prevent the development of the disease in a child or a sibling of a person with IBD.

This is primarily because we do not know exactly what triggers the development of IBD in a person who is at risk. We also do not know how the possible risk factors that individuals might be exposed to will interact with their genetic makeup. Some environmental factors may be protective in individuals with a certain genetic makeup and may increase risk of disease in other individuals with another genetic makeup. An example of this is the effect of cigarette smoking, which seems to protect against the development of ulcerative colitis, whereas it may increase the risk of Crohn's disease or, possibly, make the course of disease more severe.

No Guarantees

Children of a parent with IBD are much more likely not to develop IBD in their lifetime than they are to develop the disease. In other words, the presence of a positive genetic test or genetic risk factor, such as a family history of IBD, does not equal the presence of IBD. Likewise, a negative result on the current genetic risk markers does not guarantee that IBD will not develop in the future.

Multiple Genes

By examining the patterns of IBD inheritance in families, it is clear that Crohn's disease and ulcerative colitis are not passed from parent to child in a simple or direct fashion the way that some physical characteristics, such as eye color, blood type, or some diseases (cystic fibrosis, for example) are passed on from parent to child. In those instances, a single gene is responsible for the particular characteristic or disease. In IBD, it appears that mutations of multiple genes are required to produce increased susceptibility to the disease.

Research into the genetic factors that contribute to IBD has been exploding in the past decade with several major successes. These successes will almost certainly lead to improved understanding of how IBD occurs and, with time, may lead to improved treatments or preventive therapy.

Is My Family at Risk?

If you or a family member has IBD, the fact that certain genes, when abnormal or altered, may lead to an increased risk of developing IBD is of some interest, particularly if such knowledge ultimately leads to more effective treatment, prevention, or even cure. However, what you really want to know is, what is the risk to other family members and is there a way to predict who might develop IBD?

The risk of developing IBD is highest in first-degree relatives (brothers, sisters, parents, and children) of an affected individual. This risk to family members is higher if the person has Crohn's disease rather than ulcerative colitis. The risks described below are estimated based upon the observed frequency of Crohn's disease and ulcerative colitis within families and should not be considered necessarily exact.

Genetic Testing

Unfortunately, genetic testing for IBD is not yet sensitive enough to be used as a routine tool to predict the development of disease. Even if predictive tests were more sensitive, the results may not be valuable for treating the disease for several reasons.

Possible False Symptoms

A positive genetic test in someone with a family history may make that person or family members more vigilant in watching for early signs of disease. This may unnecessarily increase anxiety around the occurrence of symptoms that are in no way related to IBD.

Genetic Counseling

Any predictive genetic testing for any disorder should ideally be accompanied by counseling from an expert physician or genetic counselor *before* the test is made. Information derived from the test may have no value for predicting disease or treating the disorder in an individual. However, this information could potentially be used by insurance companies to deny coverage or by employers to limit employment opportunities.

Possible Unnecessary Treatment

We also do not know if earlier detection of disease, even before symptoms have begun, will allow more effective treatment of acute symptoms or prevention of long-term disease complications. Early treatment of the disease, before symptoms have begun, may produce more harm than good, unless that treatment is highly effective and very safe. Current treatments for IBD are either minimally effective or are more effective but with the cost of potential side effects, some of which may be quite serious.

Despite the reservations surrounding genetic testing, it is quite likely that some people with a family history of IBD and even some without any family history will wish to have genetic testing where it is made available. Although we do not know for certain if early treatment is of benefit, many people with positive genetic tests, even without signs or symptoms of disease, will choose to receive treatment. In a survey of IBD patients, a large percentage said they would choose to have genetic testing for their children, even if a positive test had a very low likelihood of predicting disease.

Pharmacogenomics

Where genetic testing may be more widely used, at least in the next few years, is for predicting complications and the course of the disease. Genetic testing may also prove to be valuable in treating the disease, especially in choosing effective medications. This involves the science of pharmacogenomics.

Pharmacogenomics is the use of genetic testing to predict various aspects of response — both good and bad — to medications. For example, genetic testing may predict who will respond positively to a given medication and who will likely develop side effects and thus may not be a good candidate for a given medication or may require closer monitoring.

In IBD treatment, this may occur with the use of the immune modulator drugs azathioprine and 6-mercaptopurine. The way these drugs are metabolized (broken down) in the body is determined, to a large extent, by genetic factors. Most people break the drug down into inactive by-products at roughly the same rate. However, about 10% of people break the drug down slightly more slowly, and about 1% or less break the drug down very slowly. With slow drug metabolism, there may be higher levels of the active drug in the body for the same dose. Levels of the drug that are too high tend to produce toxicity to the bone marrow, resulting in production of fewer white blood cells and the possibility of infection.

> **Tailored Treatments**
>
> As we become more knowledgeable about the way various drug therapies work and the genes that determine their ability to improve disease symptoms or produce side effects, we may be able to develop treatments that can be tailored specifically for individuals based upon their genetic profile.

With the information
gained from these genetic
associations and an
understanding of how
protein products normally
act in the body, it is
possible to begin to piece
together the complex
processes that occur in
people suffering from IBD.

Metabolism of these drugs is determined by the level of the TPMT enzyme in the bloodstream, which, in turn, is determined, to a large extent, by a specific genetic factor that can be detected through blood tests. By testing for the level of this enzyme in the blood, it may be possible to predict who is at risk for complications that occur as a result of high drug levels in the body. In this case, these drugs are often best avoided or, if used, given at much lower doses than would normally be used to treat IBD.

Unified Theory

Research has found no single cause or pathway to Crohn's disease or ulcerative colitis. Prevailing wisdom suggests that inflammatory bowel disease typically occurs in a genetically susceptible person when triggered by environmental factors.

- Someone may have inherited this susceptibility without anyone else being affected in the family. Probably, a specific combination of genetic changes or mutations comes together in an individual that, in turn, leads to this increased disease susceptibility.
- In a person with this inherited susceptibility, there may be some type of environmental exposure that, if present at sufficient levels for a sufficient period of time, will trigger uncontrolled intestinal inflammation.

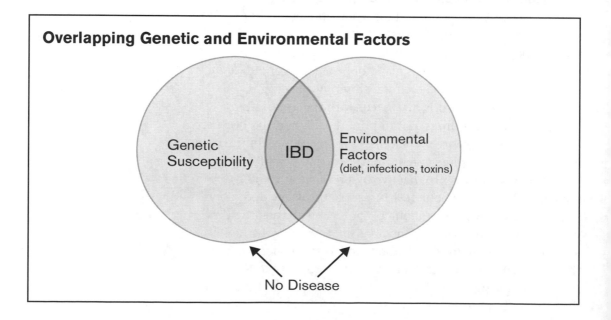

Overlapping Genetic and Environmental Factors

Genetic
Susceptibility

IBD

Environmental
Factors
(diet, infections, toxins)

No Disease

- The timing of this exposure, relative to the person's age, stage of development, and presence of other environmental factors, may be critical in the process leading to disease. Alternatively, there may be protective factors that, if a susceptible individual is not exposed to, will lead to a greater likelihood of developing of IBD.
- In humans, IBD can sometimes be successfully treated with antibiotic therapy. Antibiotic treatment is not necessarily killing a disease-causing bacteria; rather, it is changing the balance or composition of the normal intestinal bacterial population.

Based upon these observations, you could imagine a situation in which a genetically susceptible individual develops long-lasting uncontrolled intestinal inflammation in the presence of certain normal intestinal bacteria and possibly other environmental and dietary factors. Once initiated in a genetically susceptible person, it may not be possible to shut down or decrease the uncontrolled inflammation completely. As a result, the intestine is damaged, and the symptoms of IBD become evident. In a person who is not genetically susceptible, the inflammation can be kept at levels that are sufficient to protect against infections or other outside attackers, but not so high that it would cause excessive damage to the lining of the intestine.

Intestinal Bacteria
Among environmental factors, there is considerable evidence to support the role of intestinal bacteria as being critical to the development of IBD. In almost every animal model of IBD where the role of intestinal bacteria has been studied, IBD does not develop when the experimental animals are raised in an environment that does not allow them to develop normal intestinal bacteria. If intestinal bacteria are introduced into the animal or into the environment, the animal then develops IBD.

Implications for Treatment

By following these lines of inquiry and remaining open to new discoveries, we may soon be able to identify all the pieces of this complex puzzle and, ultimately, put them together to provide a complete picture of the causes of IBD. In the meantime, there is much we can do to manage this disease successfully with diet, counseling, medications, and surgery.

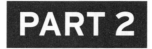

PART 2

MANAGING INFLAMMATORY BOWEL DISEASE

CHAPTER 5

Dietary Strategies for Managing IBD

Julie Robers and A. Hillary Steinhart

CASE STUDY Sabrina

Sabrina is an active 24-year-old woman who was diagnosed with Crohn's disease last year. She works during the day, but still finds time to participate in her favorite team sports and to meet with friends for dinner and movies. For the past month, Sabrina has noticed cramps and occasional abdominal pain after eating. At her friend's last barbecue, she ate steak, baked potato, and corn on the cob, but soon after, she had to leave the gathering early as a result of symptoms of abdominal bloating, cramping, and pain.

Because this had never happened before when she had eaten out, Sabrina decided to find out what she could do to improve her situation. She searched the Internet for information on any connections between diet and Crohn's disease, especially foods that might trigger flares in her disease. Friends and family offered plenty of advice about what foods she should avoid. Sabrina tried eliminating all vegetables and many fruits. She cut out red meat and dairy just in case. However, she began to lose weight quickly, enjoyed eating less, and started to stay away from get-togethers because she disliked the questions about why she was eating differently. Her cramps and pain continued despite her best efforts, so Sabrina decided it was time to make an appointment with her doctor for help.

Sabrina's health-care team provided medical therapy and answered her questions. She learned that foods don't cause or cure IBD, and that when she ate some foods, such as corn and potato skins, her symptoms worsened because these foods are difficult to digest. She was advised to follow a low-fiber diet and gradually return to her regular diet once her disease flare and symptoms resolved.

Sabrina still notices she is sensitive to some foods if they are gas-producing or she doesn't chew them well. She also understands that this type of food sensitivity is common to many people, not just those living with IBD.

Reliable Information

Nutrition is a topic of high priority not only for people living with Crohn's disease and ulcerative colitis, but also for their family and friends. Perhaps you have been diagnosed with IBD and are wondering if your current diet is appropriate. Maybe your spouse or child has been diagnosed and you are questioning if the usual foods you buy at the grocery store can still be part of your family's diet. Or maybe you've been living with IBD for a long time but are still afraid to try new foods. How can you find the answers to your questions and, at the same time, feel confident that the information you find is reliable?

Nutrition plays an important role in the management of IBD by maintaining general health during times of disease activity and during times of remission. Diet can also help with symptom management during disease flares. A person's nutritional status affects important physiological processes, such as immunity and wound healing, and, as a result, can contribute to the prevention of long-term complications. Our diet also contributes to our quality of life. Eating good-tasting food that is healthy for you should be your dietary goal, even if you have IBD symptoms. While good nutrition does not cure IBD and while, with certain exceptions, nutritional therapy does not always control disease flares, nutrition is important for health maintenance and symptom management.

Diet Studies

Diet has been studied as a possible cause of Crohn's disease and ulcerative colitis and as a possible treatment for these conditions. Although no one dietary factor has been identified as a cause of IBD, certain dietary factors could possibly play a role in triggering the disease in genetically susceptible individuals or triggering a disease flare in someone who already has the disease. These factors have not been identified, and no one diet has been proven to cure IBD. Specific foods have been identified as items to avoid in managing some symptoms.

Q **Where can I find good dietary advice?**

A Your family doctor or gastrointestinal specialist may refer you to a registered dietitian (RD) for specific dietary advice in managing your symptoms. Registered dietitians are nutrition experts in food science who have completed a university education, as well as a nationally accredited internship program. The title "Registered Dietitian" is protected in Canada under the regulated health professionals acts, whereas the title "nutritionist" has no minimum qualifications in Canada. Similar restrictions on the use of the title "Registered Dietitian" apply in the United States.

This means that a dietitian is accountable to the public for providing reliable and safe information. Dietitians are professionals qualified to consult, assess, and evaluate nutritional status and to provide advice for preventing and treating disease. Dietitians work in health care, industry, research, and government. Look for the initials behind the professional's name: RD, RDN, P.Dt., Dt.P., and R.Dt.

Q **Did something I ate cause my IBD?**

A If doctors or dietitians knew which foods, food components, food additives, food proteins, food preservatives, or food contaminants contribute to the development of IBD, they would be the first to warn susceptible individuals to avoid them. However, to start avoiding foods without scientific evidence of the real cause of this disease is a risky practice because it can affect your relationship with food and eating, can leave you with limited choices, and can result in serious health consequences as a result of inappropriately limiting nutrients. Well-founded nutrition advice can help you to achieve better health and prevent false hope without delaying effective strategies.

The Right Diet

Statement of Liability

This chapter contains references to products that may not be available everywhere. The intent of the information provided is to be helpful; however, there is no guarantee of results associated with the information provided. Use of brand names is for educational purposes only and does not imply endorsement.

No IBD Diet

While there is no such thing as an "IBD diet," there are many foods that affect IBD adversely or positively. There isn't any single diet that works for everyone with IBD.

Many people hear that a particular diet will help their IBD. Gaining a sense of control by changing what or how you eat can be appealing when living with an unpredictable disease. In some cases, the diet may claim to prevent disease relapse or even cure your IBD. Other diets claim to influence your immune system positively, improve digestive health, and reduce inflammation. However, just because it is in print does not mean it is true or scientifically valid.

Sometimes diets are applied to the body in a way that has not been proven or does not even make sense physiologically. It can be difficult to sort out myth from science. A persuasive author or an impressive anecdotal story of someone whose IBD responded only to the author's diet can be very impressive and may leave you with the impression that there is some merit in what the author is suggesting. However, such anecdotes may provide false hope. The money you spend should be for reliable, evidence-based strategies. If you've had difficulty figuring out the "right" diet to follow, it is probably because your experience with diet has been different from someone else's experience.

We each have different taste preferences, different tolerances (to spicy or gas-producing foods, for example), different budgets, and even different food availability, with limited food choices in remote areas. Not only are these circumstances applicable for an individual living with IBD, there could be additional dietary considerations, including transient intolerances to previously enjoyed foods and the need to restrict some foods temporarily and supplement others. Considering these factors, it makes sense that the same food can be experienced differently by different individuals. If you then add personal tolerances and our unique likes and dislikes, there could be many thousand versions of the "right" diet.

Individualized Diets

Accordingly, all nutrition care should be individualized and developed with your doctor or registered dietitian to ensure it is realistic and successful. Remember that Crohn's disease and ulcerative colitis have different disease characteristics, different disease courses, a variety of possible symptoms and possible complications, and variations in treatment regimens.

Nutrition recommendations must be balanced to avoid nutrient deficiencies and individualized to specific tastes, budgets, lifestyles, and very importantly, for specific desired functional benefits (for example, regaining weight, symptom management). The diet that considers and meets these needs is the right diet for you.

However, there are some common dietary guidelines that people with IBD could follow in an effort to manage their symptoms and improve their quality of life — and even ward off more serious complications, such as malnutrition.

Empowerment

Managing your own diet can provide a sense of control when living with an unpredictable and uncontrollable chronic disease, such as Crohn's disease and ulcerative colitis. To appreciate that your food choices help contribute to your health is an extremely powerful motivator.

Preventing Malnutrition

Diet is the key for preventing clinical malnutrition, a condition that results when there is a deficiency or imbalance of nutrients in our body. Nutrient deficiencies can result over time from a lack of overall calories (the term "calories" can be used interchangeably with "energy") or from a lack of specific nutrients, such as protein, essential fats, vitamins, minerals, or trace elements.

Malnutrition is a concern because it can affect your immune system function, leading to an increased susceptibility to infections. It also compromises your body's normal defenses against free radicals (damaging molecules produced from pollution, radiation, stress, and smoking), slows down wound healing, and can contribute to long-term complications, such as poor dental health and early bone loss leading to osteoporosis. When you are poorly nourished, the symptoms of your IBD are likely to become more severe or have a more significant impact upon you.

Malnutrition Symptoms

Malnutrition can manifest as weight loss, loss of appetite, muscle weakness (from losing muscle mass), or changes in your skin, hair, nails, gums, eyesight, or mood.

Weight Loss

The most common indicator of malnutrition is a significant loss of body weight. Often, when you are not feeling well, you have little appetite and must force yourself to eat. And often you still lose weight despite your efforts. Why does this happen? This is not simply a matter of willpower.

In Crohn's disease and ulcerative colitis, various parts of the gastrointestinal tract become inflamed, and although the inflammation occurs primarily at a local level (the bowel tissue), it can also occur at a whole body, or "systemic," level. Systemic inflammation results from inflammatory molecules (proteins called cytokines), which are produced in the inflamed intestine, but which circulate throughout the body. It is the effect of one or more of these cytokines that can lead to a loss of appetite.

Anorexia is one malnutrition risk factor that, along with other symptoms, such as gastrointestinal intolerance, altered taste, and dietary eliminations (food phobias and dependencies), can lead to inadequate intake. Other risk factors for malnutrition include increased nutrient requirements, malabsorption of nutrients, and increased losses of electrolytes, minerals, trace elements, and proteins. These factors can lead to malnutrition in individuals with IBD, but this doesn't mean that you will develop these symptoms or complications just because you have IBD. Also keep in mind that some are specific to either Crohn's disease or ulcerative colitis.

Treatment for Malnutrition

To determine if you are malnourished, health-care professionals will evaluate your symptoms and signs, medical history, height and weight trends, diet history, social and economic circumstances, medications, and laboratory tests. Although there are several complicated formulas that have been developed to evaluate nutritional status and nutritional risk, most physicians and dietitians can answer these questions quite easily. An appropriate nutrition plan can then be created to help manage your illness and achieve your desired health outcomes.

Your nutrition plan could include counseling for diet modifications or implementing specialized nutrition therapies. These could include supplementation with nutritional products, replacement of vitamins and minerals, provision of enteral nutrition (liquid nutrition formula delivered using a feeding tube into the stomach or small intestine), or provision of parenteral nutrition (intravenous nutrition infused through a special intravenous line).

Malnutrition Risk Factors

1. Inadequate Intake of Nutrients

- **Anorexia**
  - Decreased oral intake of food and beverages
  - Inability to tolerate solid foods and a prolonged period consuming low-calorie and protein fluids

- **Gastrointestinal intolerance**
  - Nausea, vomiting, diarrhea, rectal urgency, cramping, bloating, pain, obstructive symptoms, pain with swallowing

- **Altered taste**
  - Side effect from some medications

- **Dietary eliminations**
  - Food phobias, food intolerances, diet experimentation
  - Dependencies (e.g., substituting alcohol for nutritious foods)

2. Increased Nutrient Requirements

- **Higher metabolic rate**
  - Stress response and inflammation, infection, wound healing, fever, catabolic (breakdown) effects from steroids
  - Increased requirements for growth (children and adolescents)
  - Repletion (building) of body tissue stores of muscle and fat

3. Malabsorption of Nutrients

- **Decreased absorptive surface**
  - Active disease affecting bowel surface
  - Multiple surgical resections

- **Nutrient bypass**
  - Fistula
  - Surgical

- **Drug interference**

- **Bile salt deficiency**

- **Bacterial overgrowth in small intestine**

4. Increased Losses (electrolytes, minerals, trace elements, protein)

- **Diarrhea**

- **Fistula**

- **Blood loss**

Eating Well with Canada's Food Guide

Recommended Number of *Food Guide Servings* per Day

	Children			Teens		Adults			
Age in Years	2-3	4-8	9-13	14-18		19-50		51+	
Sex	Girls and Boys			Females	Males	Females	Males	Females	Males
Vegetables and Fruit	4	5	6	7	8	7-8	8-10	7	7
Grain Products	3	4	6	6	7	6-7	8	6	7
Milk and Alternatives	2	2	3-4	3-4	3-4	2	2	3	3
Meat and Alternatives	1	1	1-2	2	3	2	3	2	3

What is One Food Guide Serving?
Look at the examples below.

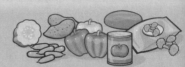

Fresh, frozen or canned vegetables
125 mL (½ cup)

Bread
1 slice (35 g)

Bagel
½ bagel (45 g)

Milk or powdered milk (reconstituted)
250 mL (1 cup)

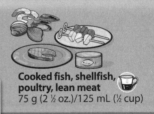

Cooked fish, shellfish, poultry, lean meat
75 g (2 ½ oz.)/125 mL (½ cup)

The chart above shows how many Food Guide Servings you need from each of the four food groups every day.

Having the amount and type of food recommended and following the tips in *Canada's Food Guide* will help:

• Meet your needs for vitamins, minerals and other nutrients.
• Reduce your risk of obesity, type 2 diabetes, heart disease, certain types of cancer and osteoporosis.
• Contribute to your overall health and vitality.

For a full guide, please contact Health Canada or visit their website.

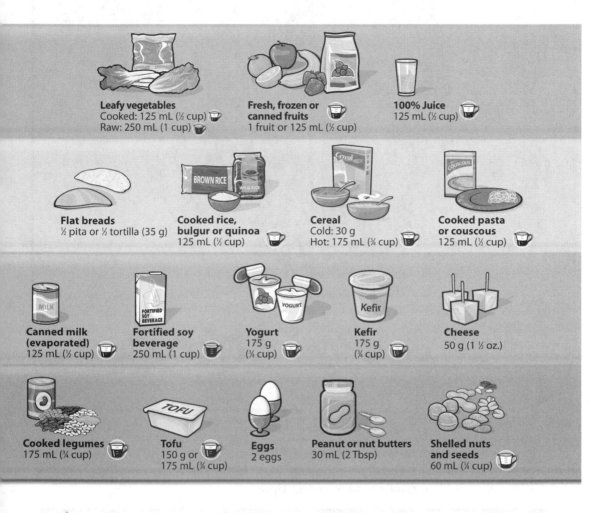

Leafy vegetables
Cooked: 125 mL (½ cup)
Raw: 250 mL (1 cup)

Fresh, frozen or canned fruits
1 fruit or 125 mL (½ cup)

100% Juice
125 mL (½ cup)

Flat breads
½ pita or ½ tortilla (35 g)

Cooked rice, bulgur or quinoa
125 mL (½ cup)

Cereal
Cold: 30 g
Hot: 175 mL (¾ cup)

Cooked pasta or couscous
125 mL (½ cup)

Canned milk (evaporated)
125 mL (½ cup)

Fortified soy beverage
250 mL (1 cup)

Yogurt
175 g
(¾ cup)

Kefir
175 g
(¾ cup)

Cheese
50 g (1 ½ oz.)

Cooked legumes
175 mL (¾ cup)

Tofu
150 g or
175 mL (¾ cup)

Eggs
2 eggs

Peanut or nut butters
30 mL (2 Tbsp)

Shelled nuts and seeds
60 mL (¼ cup)

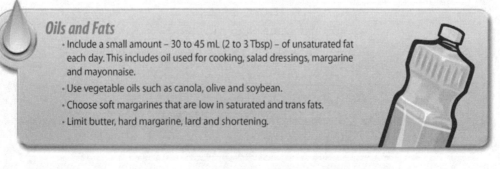

Oils and Fats

- Include a small amount – 30 to 45 mL (2 to 3 Tbsp) – of unsaturated fat each day. This includes oil used for cooking, salad dressings, margarine and mayonnaise.
- Use vegetable oils such as canola, olive and soybean.
- Choose soft margarines that are low in saturated and trans fats.
- Limit butter, hard margarine, lard and shortening.

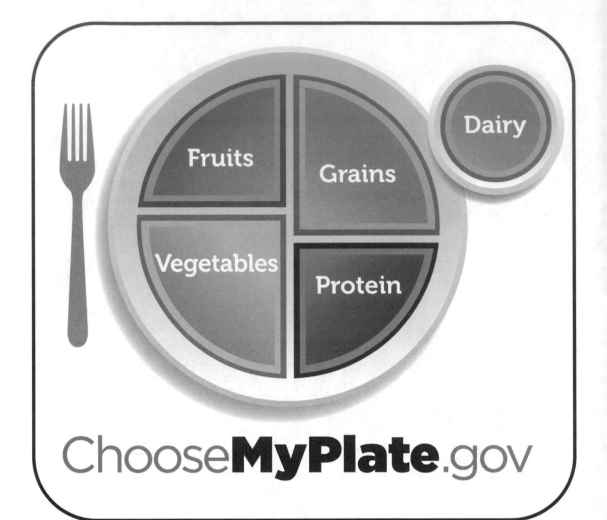

Choose**MyPlate**.gov

Balancing Calories
- Enjoy your food, but eat less.
- Avoid oversized portions.

Foods to Increase
- Make half your plate fruits and vegetables.
- Make at least half your grains whole grains.
- Switch to fat-free or low-fat (1%) milk.

Foods to Reduce
- Compare sodium in foods like soup, bread, and frozen meals and choose the foods with lower numbers.
- Drink water instead of sugary drinks.

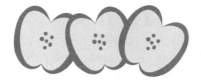

Vegetarian food guide rainbow

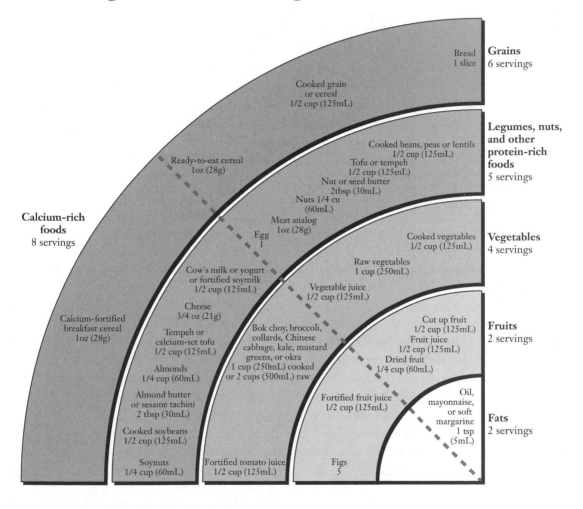

Grains
6 servings

Bread
1 slice

Cooked grain
or cereal
1/2 cup (125mL)

**Legumes, nuts,
and other
protein-rich
foods**
5 servings

Cooked beans, peas or lentils
1/2 cup (125mL)

Tofu or tempeh
1/2 cup (125mL)

Nut or seed butter
2tbsp (30mL)

Nuts 1/4 cu
(60mL)

Meat analog
1oz (28g)

Egg
1

Ready-to-eat cereal
1oz (28g)

**Calcium-rich
foods**
8 servings

Cow's milk or yogurt
or fortified soymilk
1/2 cup (125mL)

Cheese
3/4 oz (21g)

Tempeh or
calcium-set tofu
1/2 cup (125mL)

Almonds
1/4 cup (60mL)

Almond butter
or sesame tachini
2 tbsp (30mL)

Cooked soybeans
1/2 cup (125mL)

Calcium-fortified
breakfast cereal
1oz (28g)

Soynuts
1/4 cup (60mL)

Vegetables
4 servings

Cooked vegetables
1/2 cup (125mL)

Raw vegetables
1 cup (250mL)

Vegetable juice
1/2 cup (125mL)

Bok choy, broccoli,
collards, Chinese
cabbage, kale, mustard
greens, or okra
1 cup (250mL) cooked
or 2 cups (500mL) raw

Fortified tomato juice
1/2 cup (125mL)

Fruits
2 servings

Cut up fruit
1/2 cup (125mL)

Fruit juice
1/2 cup (125mL)

Dried fruit
1/4 cup (60mL)

Fortified fruit juice
1/2 cup (125mL)

Figs
5

Fats
2 servings

Oil,
mayonnaise,
or soft
margarine
1 tsp
(5mL)

Source: Figure 2 - A new food guide for North American vegetarians. Messina V, Melina V, Mangels AR.
Can Diet Pract Res. 2003; 64(2):82. (www.dietitians.ca/news/downloads/Vegetarian_Food_Guide_for_NA.pdf)
Copyright 2003. Dietitians of Canada. Used with permission.

**Dietitians of Canada
Les diététistes du Canada**

Diet Modifications

If your IBD is under control and you live relatively symptom free, there is no need to restrict foods or follow a special diet. Just follow the United States Department of Agriculture (USDA) MyPlate Food Guidance System or Canada's Food Guide. The Dietitians of Canada have also created a Vegetarian Food Guide Rainbow. These reliable diet guides emphasize eating a wide variety of foods that provide the multitude of nutrients your body needs. The key is to select a variety of foods from all food groups in the recommended amounts.

However, if you are experiencing acute disease activity, you may find it helpful to modify your regular diet to help minimize gastrointestinal symptoms, such as cramping, bloating, gas, and diarrhea. Remember that diet plays an important role in maintaining nutritional status, but also in helping with symptom management. It is of utmost importance that dietary changes do not compromise nutritional status or well-being. This means maintaining weight and energy intake levels, continuing to enjoy eating, and participating in social situations involving food.

Q Do I need to modify my diet?

A By asking yourself, your doctor, and your dietitian the following questions, you can determine what dietary modifications, if any, you might require:
- What is the status of my disease?
- What symptoms am I currently experiencing?
- If my disease is active, what part or parts of my bowel are affected? What nutrients are usually absorbed in this location?
- Are there any complications from my disease that I should also consider – osteoporosis or strictures (narrowed bowel from scar tissue), for example?
- What effect does my treatment have on nutrient requirements?
- Do my medications interact with nutrients?
- Has surgery affected the amount of remaining bowel available for absorption?

Diet Modification Goals

There are specific goals for diet modifications to address not only symptom management, but also to help achieve better physical and emotional health. For instance, there can be a feeling of social isolation when your food choices are limited or you need to ask for special accommodations when eating away from home. Sometimes you just want to feel "normal" like everyone else.

Diet Modification Goals

1. ## Normalize bowel function
   - Decrease stool frequency
   - Increase stool consistency

2. ## Minimize GI intolerance symptoms
   - Reduce gas, bloating, cramping, pain
   - Reduce obstruction risk

3. ## Maintain hydration and electrolyte balance

4. ## Maintain or improve nutritional status
   - Prevent further weight loss (or weight gain if applicable)
   - Improve functional status
   - Supplement with specific nutrients if indicated

5. ## Continue or resume social participation and enjoyment
   - Normalize diet with time
   - Improve relationship with food

Elimination Diets

Elimination diets are popular in the diet industry, and complementary and alternative medicine practitioners may also take this approach to treatment. This type of diet significantly restricts or excludes one or more foods or major food groups. Common examples of exclusions include dairy, wheat, red meat, yeast, and refined sugars. If you choose to follow an elimination diet, be sure to consider the potential side effects.

Side Effects

Consequences of following exclusionary diets over the long term — that is, for more than a few weeks — include possible development of nutrient deficiencies, weight loss, malnutrition, food phobias or obsessions, and a loss of enjoyment of eating. If major food groups are avoided, be sure to speak with a dietitian to learn about alternative foods or supplements for the excluded nutrients.

Exclusion Diet Value

The value of exclusion diets has not been scientifically proven in IBD. In studies where suspected foods were excluded, individuals didn't experience disease relapse upon reintroduction of the excluded foods.

There is also a psychological danger with elimination diets. Following a diet that claims to control your IBD can contribute to a feeling of being somehow responsible or guilty if your disease becomes active again. Some people feel they may have cheated on the diet because they had difficulty following it exactly, and they are now responsible for their disease coming back. There is no evidence to support this. This type of internalization of responsibility is destructive and takes strength away during a time when it is difficult enough to live with IBD.

If you still feel it is important to try this approach, be sure to set a timeline for evaluating and stopping the dietary eliminations.

Lactose-Restricted Diets

<table>
<tr><td>

Lactose Intolerance

Lactose intolerance is when your body cannot adequately digest the milk sugar lactose.

</td></tr>
</table>

Is there ever a time when it may be appropriate to reduce consumption or avoid a particular food group? When it comes to dairy products, the answer is yes. Delicious but dangerous is a slogan to apply to dairy products if you have IBD. While dairy products are tasty and provide important nutrients, such as protein and calcium, there are specific situations where it may be difficult to digest the primary sugar in milk.

Unless you have a true milk allergy (immune reaction to the protein in milk), there is no danger from eating dairy products. This type of allergy is relatively uncommon. Dairy products do not cause IBD and generally do not result in flares, but you may experience uncomfortable symptoms if you have lactose intolerance and you drink milk or eat dairy products.

Lactase Deficiency

Lactose is the principal carbohydrate in dairy products. It is a disaccharide, meaning that it is a larger molecule made up of two smaller sugar molecules, which are the monosaccharides glucose and galactose. An enzyme called lactase in our small intestine is responsible for breaking lactose into glucose and galactose, which are then easily absorbed.

If there is not enough lactase enzyme available to break down lactose into its two smaller sugars, the result is undigested lactose traveling through the small intestine to the large intestine (colon). This is why lactose intolerance can also be correctly called lactase deficiency.

Lactose Intolerance Symptoms

The classic symptoms of lactose intolerance result from undigested lactose traveling through the small bowel and drawing water by osmosis into the bowel, which causes bloating. When the undigested lactose reaches the colon, bacteria ferment it, producing further bloating, cramping, gas, and diarrhea. Symptoms vary among individuals, but typically appear within 30 minutes to several hours after ingestion.

Q How do I know if I might be susceptible to lactose intolerance?

A There are at least two possible factors involved in causing lactose intolerance: genetics and acquired factors.

Genetics: The most common cause of lactose intolerance in adults has to do with genetics. There is a natural decline in lactase production as we age (genetically determined rate). This natural decline in the amount of lactase enzyme present on the surface of the small bowel occurs as people age and leads to progressive lactose intolerance (this is called primary lactase deficiency).

Although everyone experiences a decrease in lactase production over their lifetime, the rate at which this occurs is different for different ethnic groups. Certain ethnic groups have a genetic predisposition to lactase deficiency, including individuals of African, Jewish, and Asian descent. Conversely, individuals of Scandinavian and Northern European descent have the lowest prevalence of lactose intolerance. North Americans of similar ancestry have demonstrated similar prevalence rates.

Acquired Lactase Deficiency: External factors can sometimes result in a deficiency in the amount of lactase enzyme available on the small bowel surface (called secondary lactase deficiency). This may occur following medical treatment (for example, chemotherapy, radiation, or multiple small bowel resections), in malnutrition, or from active small intestinal disease, such as Crohn's disease. Once the disease or injury resolves, lactase production resumes and digestion of lactose usually improves, but not always.

Lactose Intolerance Testing

A hydrogen breath test, which involves drinking a test dose of lactose, can help to determine if you are lactose intolerant. If a person has lactase deficiency, the unabsorbed lactose will be fermented by colonic bacteria and hydrogen gas will be formed. Some of this hydrogen gas is absorbed into your bloodstream and breathed out through the lungs, where it can be measured in your breath.

If you have a hydrogen breath test, be sure to ask what dose of lactose you were tested with. Depending on the lab, doses can range anywhere from 12.5 g of lactose (equivalent to 1 cup/250 mL of milk) to 50 g of lactose (equivalent to 4 cups/1 L of milk). Many people can drink one glass of milk without difficulty, but would rarely drink a quart or liter of milk at one time, so the relevance (applicability to your daily life) of the test depends on the dose administered.

Dairy Reduction

Fortunately, many individuals who develop lactose intolerance can still consume small amounts of dairy, just not as much as before. This is called a dose-dependent effect. In these cases, eliminating dairy products is not necessary, just a reduction in the amount of dairy product taken at one time. Interestingly, some people can gradually increase their tolerance to dairy. This has nothing to do with the amount of lactase enzyme they have, but rather their gastrointestinal bacteria are able to adapt to the lactose load.

Lactose Ladder

This lactose ladder lists dairy products and their lactose content. You can start climbing from the bottom (lowest lactose-containing foods) and make your way as far up to the top (higher lactose-containing foods) as you can tolerate.

Source	Serving	Lactose (grams)
Skim milk	1 cup (250 mL)	13.3
2% milk	1 cup (250 mL)	11.6
Yogurt (with probiotics to reduce lactose)	1/2 cup (125 mL)	6.3-9.5
Ice cream	1/2 cup (125 mL)	4.9
Cottage cheese	1/2 cup (125 mL)	2.9–3.9
Cream cheese	1 oz (30 g)	0.7
Cream (whipping, half & half)	1 tbsp (15 mL)	0.6
Dry curd cottage cheese	1/2 cup (125 mL)	0.5
Cheese (Cheddar, Gouda, blue, Colby)	1 oz (30 g)	0.5–0.8
Parmesan cheese	1 tbsp (15 mL), grated	0.2
Cheese (camembert, limburger)	1 oz (30 g)	0.1
Butter	1 tsp (5 mL)	Trace

Hidden Lactose

There are also hidden sources of lactose in foods. If you are severely lactose intolerant, you will need to avoid all sources of lactose. Lactose can be added as a filler in some medications and some foods (for example, processed meats, gravies, breads, cereals, salad dressings, breakfast drinks, cake mixes, margarine). Lactose may also be present if the label lists added milk solids, whey, curds, butter, or cheese flavor. Casein does not contain lactose. Be sure to read food labels for hidden sources.

Q **Should I try reducing or avoiding lactose?**

A Controversy exists regarding the clinical prevalence of secondary lactase deficiency in IBD. This is because the lactose intolerance studies have not always taken age or ethnicity into account (factors we know affect the amount of lactase enzyme). Lactose intolerance may be more common in IBD; however, this is not definitive. Often doctors will ask a person to restrict dairy in the diet temporarily to determine how the disease is responding to treatment and to prevent misdiagnosis of any lactose intolerance symptoms as disease activity symptoms. Bloating, cramping, and diarrhea could be misdiagnosed as ongoing IBD symptoms.

If your symptoms improve while avoiding lactose, then a temporary restriction is right for you. If not, it is important not to restrict dairy from your diet unnecessarily. When your flare improves, it is worthwhile increasing dairy in your diet again. This is especially true if you tolerated dairy products before your flare or if you miss eating dairy products.

Ileostomy

If you have an ileostomy and are lactose intolerant, you can still eat dairy products. The undigested lactose will reach the ileostomy pouch instead of being fermented in the colon (which may have been surgically removed). The ileostomy pouch may develop more gas (from the bacteria in the stool), but it will not give you the same symptoms of cramping, bloating, and diarrhea.

Calcium Sources

Dairy products are important sources of calcium, and some of these products are fortified with vitamin D. Calcium and vitamin D are critical for good bone and tooth health (other important nutrients for bone health include phosphorus, magnesium, and fluoride). A diet that includes adequate amounts of these nutrients is one important factor to help prevent bone loss (osteopenia) and development of osteoporosis.

Increased Calcium Need

Individuals with IBD are at risk of osteoporosis. If you chose to restrict dairy products in your diet, you will need to consider increasing your calcium and perhaps vitamin D intake from other sources.

Other Food Sources of Calcium

You may limit dairy because of lactose intolerance or avoid it entirely for other reasons, such as taste, ethics, allergy, or cultural or religious traditions. Regardless of the reason, the challenge is to get the key nutrients provided by this food group in other ways. Calcium from dairy products is better absorbed than calcium in many other foods.

Enzyme Supplements

Another strategy for consuming adequate calcium when you are lactose intolerant is to use a commercial lactase enzyme product to break down lactose. These are available as tablets or as liquid drops in most pharmacies.

Q How do you know if I am getting enough calcium?

A Recommended amounts (known as Dietary Reference Intakes, or DRIs) for nutrients are based on age and gender. In adults, the range for calcium is generally 1000 to 1300 mg per day, depending on your age, gender, if you are pregnant, if you have osteoporosis, or if you have any condition that affects metabolism or absorption of calcium and vitamin D (check with your health-care team to find the specific amount recommended for you). In clinical practice, doctors advise amounts that also take bone health and medication use (for example, steroid use) into consideration.

Lactose-free products (milk, yogurt, ice cream) will contain the same amount of calcium (and the same amount of vitamin D, in the case of milk) as their lactose-containing versions (only the lactose content has changed). The absorption of calcium from plant-based sources is reduced due to compounds called oxalates (found in dark green leafy vegetables, such as spinach and beet greens) and phytates (found in whole grains, nuts, seeds, and legumes). These foods have decreased bioavailability of calcium because the oxalates and phytates bind to minerals, such as calcium, thus interfering with absorption.

If you suspect you are not meeting the recommended amounts for calcium or vitamin D, consult with your doctor or a registered dietitian.

Dairy Sources of Calcium

In order to get enough calcium, it is recommended that adults consume two to four servings of milk products per day. This table lists common lactose-containing sources of calcium (milligrams of calcium rounded) approximated to usual serving sizes.

Source	Serving	Calcium (mg)
Cow's milk (skim, 1%, 2%, whole, chocolate, buttermilk) and goat's milk	1 cup (250 mL)	285–330
Evaporated milk, partly skimmed	1/2 cup (125 mL)	350
Powdered milk	6 tbsp (90 mL), dry	320
Cream soup (made with milk)	1 cup (250 mL)	175–190
Pudding (made with milk)	1/2 cup (125 mL)	105–165
Yogurt (plain or flavored or fruit bottom)	3/4 cup (175 mL)	215–325
Yogurt drink	3/4 cup (175 mL)	185
Frozen yogurt	1/2 cup (125 mL)	150
Ice cream or ice milk	1/2 cup (125 mL)	80–90
Sour cream (non-fat)	1/2 cup (125 mL)	225
Cottage cheese (1% or 2%)	1/2 cup (125 mL)	70–85
Processed cheese: thin slice thick slice	2 slices (1 1/2 oz/42 g) 2 slices (2 oz/62 g)	255 385
Cheese (soft) • Brie • Camembert • Ricotta (part skim) Cheese (hard) • Parmesan cheese • Cheddar, Gouda, Colby, Edam, brick, Swiss cheese • Feta cheese • Mozzarella	 1 3/4 oz (50 g) 1 3/4 oz (50 g) 1/2 cup (125 mL) 3 tbsp (45 mL), grated 1 3/4 oz (50 g) 1 3/4 oz (50 g) 1 3/4 oz (50 g)	 90 195 340 260 350–480 255 270

Supplements

If you don't think you can improve your intake from food and beverages, consider calcium supplements with vitamin D and discuss this with your doctor. There may be times when your doctor recommends supplements in addition to foods. There are many forms of calcium supplements to choose from — pills, effervescent tablets, chewable tablets, and "soft chews" in multiple flavors. Be sure to choose calcium supplements that also contain vitamin D.

Alternative Food Sources of Calcium

Consider the following suggestions for alternative food and supplement sources of calcium (milligrams of calcium rounded).

Source	Serving	Calcium (mg)
Fortified soy milk (absorption of calcium may be slightly less than cow's milk)	1 cup (250 mL)	300
Fortified orange juice	1 cup (250 mL)	300
Orange	1 (medium)	50
Fortified rice beverage	1 cup (250 mL)	300
Fortified plant-based beverages — almond, hemp, coconut, cashew "milk" (nut beverages do not contain the same nutrients as cow's milk or soy milk)	1 cup (250 mL)	Varies (read label)
Tofu (soft) set with calcium sulphate	$\frac{1}{3}$ cup (75 mL)	150 (check label)
Nuts and seeds • Almonds • Brazil nuts (dried) • Sesame seeds (whole dried)	 1 oz (30 g), 24 nuts 1 oz (30 g), 8 medium nuts 1 tbsp (15 mL)	 75 50 88
Legumes (cooked) • Baked or refried beans • Chickpeas • Red kidney beans • Navy, white, soybeans	 1 cup (250 mL) 1 cup (250 mL) 1 cup (250 mL) 1 cup (250 mL)	 130–165 85 50 90–200
Vegetables (cooked) • Spinach • Broccoli • Bok choy, kale, Swiss chard • Collard greens	 $\frac{1}{2}$ cup (125 mL) $\frac{1}{2}$ cup (125 mL) $\frac{1}{2}$ cup (125 mL) $\frac{1}{2}$ cup (25 mL)	 130 40–50 50–105 180
Pink or sockeye salmon (with bones)	$\frac{1}{2}$ can ($\frac{2}{3}$ cup/175 mL)	225–240
Sardines (with bones)	$\frac{1}{2}$ can (2 oz/55 g), 4 pieces	200
Blackstrap molasses	1 tsp (5 mL)	60
Figs	6 (dried)	150

Optimal Dose

On the label, look at the "elemental" calcium content — that is, the calcium available to your body. Split calcium dosages so that you are taking no more than 500 mg elemental calcium at any one time in order to get maximal absorption. For some forms of calcium, take the supplements with meals. Calcium carbonate, for example, requires stomach acid for absorption, whereas calcium citrate or gluconate do not.

Discuss the safest sources of calcium supplements with your pharmacist. Dolomite or bone meal, for example, are most contaminated by lead; oyster shell or shellfish sources may pass government standards; and calcium citrate and refined calcium carbonates are considered lowest in lead content.

Vitamin D

Vitamin D helps your body absorb calcium. Interestingly, vitamin D is a hormone that our bodies make when sunlight shines on our skin (sunlight provides ultraviolet radiation for the body to convert vitamin D to an active form). In northern latitudes of North America and Europe, the reduced sunshine and angle of the sun in winter months results in less vitamin D manufactured by the skin. Similarly, if individuals have dark skin (more pigmentation), are housebound or institutionalized, or wear sunscreen at all times when outdoors, they are also at risk of not getting enough vitamin D. Generally speaking, if you have 10 to 15 minutes of sunlight exposure (face, arms, hands, without sunscreen) twice a week, you are probably getting enough vitamin D. What can influence this estimate is your geographic location, the time of year, your age, and your skin color.

Optimal Dose

Because of the factors that interfere with our ability to get enough vitamin D, select items in our food supply are fortified with vitamin D. The combination of sun exposure, food sources, and supplements is thought to allow most North Americans to meet their vitamin D needs. The importance of vitamin D relates to its well-established positive role with respect to building and maintaining bone health. Vitamin D has also recently been evaluated for its purported benefit of protecting against other chronic diseases, including cancer, cardiovascular disease, and diabetes. However, there has been insufficient evidence to date that a higher intake will confer these benefits.

In 2010, the Food and Nutrition Board at the Institute of Medicine (IOM), which is the health arm of the National Academy of Sciences, published revised recommendations for the recommended amount of vitamin D intake. In its report, commissioned by the Canadian and American governments, the DRI for vitamin D for adults was raised from 200 IU to 600 to 800 IU, depending on age and sex (for example, a higher amount is

Fortified?
Milk is almost always fortified with vitamin D, but not all dairy products are good sources of vitamin D. For instance, cottage cheese is not made from fortified milk, so it does not provide vitamin D. Some food manufacturers are starting to add vitamin D to some products, so just check the label.

Vitamin D Sources

Source	Serving	Vitamin D (IU)
Cow's milk	1 cup (250 mL)	90–100
Fortified soy milk or plant-based beverage	1 cup (250 mL)	90–100 (check label)
Fortified yogurt (check label)	¾ cup (175 mL)	88
Fortified orange juice	1 cup (250 mL)	100
Fortified margarine	1 tbsp (15 mL)	60
Salmon	3 oz (90 g), cooked	360–500
Mackerel	3 oz (90 g), cooked	388
Sardines	1¾ oz (50 g), canned	250
Tuna	3 oz (90 g), canned	200
Egg	1 whole (yolk)	20–25
Cod liver oil (avoid this source because it may contain contaminants, as well as high levels of vitamin A, which can weaken bones)	1 tbsp (15 mL)	1400

Note: Be sure to check whether the fortification is with the preferred form of vitamin D_3 and not vitamin D_2, which is less potent.

recommended for high-risk groups such as the elderly). There has been considerable discussion following the publication of these guidelines, and some public health organizations (for example, the Canadian Cancer Society, Canadian Pediatrics Society, and Osteoporosis Canada) have maintained recommendations for increased doses of vitamin D anywhere from 800 to 2000 IU per day.

Adults on prednisone may be advised to take 1500 mg of calcium a day and 1000 IU of vitamin D. Vitamin D above these amounts can lead to significant health problems, so it is important to discuss any supplementation with your physician.

Expensive Urine

North Americans are said to have the most expensive urine in the world, resulting from intake of excess water-soluble vitamins that are excreted in the urine.

Other Vitamin and Mineral Supplements

Replacing or supplementing nutrients other than calcium and vitamin D may be necessary if there is a problem with absorption. Absorption of nutrients can be affected by disease activity, bacterial overgrowth, loss of bowel from surgical resections, or interference from medications.

Key micronutrients

Water-soluble vitamins	Fat-soluble vitamins	Minerals	Trace elements
• Vitamin B_1 (thiamin) • Vitamin B_2 (riboflavin) • Vitamin B_3 (niacin) • Biotin • Pantothenic acid • Vitamin B_6 (pyridoxine) • Folic acid • Vitamin B_{12} (cyanocobalamin) • Vitamin C	• Vitamin A (beta-carotene is the precursor) • Vitamin D • Vitamin E • Vitamin K	• Sodium • Chloride • Potassium • Calcium • Phosphorus • Magnesium • Sulphur	• Iron • Zinc • Iodine • Selenium • Copper • Manganese • Fluoride • Chromium • Molybdenum

Nutrient Deficiency Symptoms and Supplements

Calories: In general, if you are not able to maintain a healthy weight, you may need to boost calories (calories come from macronutrients, namely carbohydrates, protein, and fat).

Protein: You may need extra protein if you are on high-dose steroids, extra protein and iron if you have ongoing blood loss, or additional protein and zinc if you have prolonged diarrhea, a wound, or a fistula affecting your small bowel.

Fat: You may need to change the amount and supplement a specific type of fat if you have extensive Crohn's disease of the ileum or have had more than 3 feet (1 m) of terminal ileum removed surgically.

Iron: If you have anemia, you might require supplementation of iron, folate, or vitamin B_{12}.

Vitamin B_{12}: You will most likely also need to replace vitamin B_{12} by injection if your disease is active in your terminal ileum or you have had large amounts of terminal ileum surgically resected at one or more operations.

Folic acid: If you are taking sulfasalazine, you will likely need to supplement folate, as this drug interferes with folate's metabolism. Note that folic acid is the correct term for a supplement of folate.

Sodium and Potassium: If you have had large bowel removed, you will need to increase fluid and electrolytes (sodium and potassium) in your diet.

Calcium and Vitamin D: If you are treated with steroids, you will probably need additional calcium and vitamin D because steroids interfere with the absorption of calcium. Another medication called Questran (also called cholestyramine) interferes with the absorption of fat-soluble vitamins, such as vitamin D.

Vitamin B_{12} Injections

Vitamin B_{12} is absorbed only in the terminal ileum (the last part of the small intestine), so if you have Crohn's disease in that region or have had surgical resection of your terminal ileum, you most likely require supplements. Vitamin B_{12} absorption is also dependent on intrinsic factor (IF), which is secreted by the stomach, so people who have had surgery to remove part of the stomach may also require vitamin B_{12} supplements. Because the terminal ileum is diseased or removed, vitamin B_{12} won't be absorbed if you take a supplement by mouth — it must be delivered by injection.

Frequently Asked Questions about Vitamin and Mineral Supplements

If you think you may need to supplement specific nutrients, talk to your doctor.

Q **Should I take a multivitamin supplement?**

A Supplements are a good idea when a major food group is eliminated. But what about taking a supplement for times when you are busy and you do not necessarily take the time to plan, shop for, prepare, or eat nutritious meals? These regular daily activities can be especially hard for someone who isn't feeling well or is lacking in energy.

The best way to determine whether you need a supplement is to identify which food groups are not well represented in your daily diet. Remember, vitamins, minerals, and trace elements are essential to your health because your body cannot synthesize them. They must be consumed from a variety of foods.

The first step is to compare your diet to the USDA MyPlate Food Guidance System or Canada's Food Guide. For each food, a particular set of nutrients and a recommended number of servings are specified. For example, the grain products are significant sources of complex carbohydrates, riboflavin, thiamin, niacin, iron, protein, magnesium, and fiber. Thus, if an individual does not choose many servings from this group, those nutrients may be lacking. This is when it is a good idea to consider a supplement for the missing nutrients. Just remember that eating the real thing is more tasty, filling, and provides more nutrient variety. A well-balanced diet, including a variety of foods, is best for good health and can usually be eaten even if you have IBD.

Q   What vitamin and mineral supplements should I take?

A   There are many brands of standard adult multivitamins with minerals, and most varieties are fine for meeting general needs. There are special versions available, which add more target nutrients (for example, prenatal versions have more iron, calcium, and folic acid, while "silver" versions add more calcium for people over 50 years old).

More does not necessarily mean better. The "mega" or "super" or "stress" doses are not usually more beneficial because any excess that is ingested is not used by your body and is simply excreted in the urine or stored in the liver or fat tissue, which can be harmful.

There are safety risks to mega-dosing, especially with fat-soluble vitamins, which are stored in our bodies and not excreted in urine. Harm from higher doses can include toxicities; masking deficiencies of other nutrients (for example, folic acid masks vitamin B_{12} deficiency); interference with body functions, such as blood clotting (for example, excess vitamin E); risk of birth defects; liver damage (for example, excess vitamin A); or risk of kidney stones (for example, excess calcium).

Q   Are vitamins and mineral supplements safe?

A   In addition to considering the appropriate dose, how do you know if the product is safe? In Canada, when choosing a supplement, look for a D.I.N. (drug identification number) or a G.P. (general product) number, which assures you that Health Canada has approved the product as safe. This way, you know that you are getting what you are paying for. Products with a D.I.N. undergo quality assurance testing to ensure standardization, safety, and effectiveness.

In the United States, vitamins and minerals (as well as botanical products and herbs) are considered "dietary supplements" under the Dietary Supplement Health and Education Act (DSHEA) of 1994. According to this act, a company is responsible for determining that the dietary supplements it makes or distributes are safe. They must also have evidence for any claims of health benefits, but they do not need approval from the Food and Drug Administration (FDA) before they market the product. The manufacturer is responsible for listing the ingredients of the supplements, but the FDA does not monitor the quality of the dietary supplements on a routine basis. Manufacturers who introduce new supplements after 1994 are required to show evidence of the safety of their product.

Liquid Calorie Supplements

During times when you feel that you cannot get enough calories, you may want to drink commercially prepared liquid supplements. There are many different brand names, varieties, and flavors. Most are lactose free.

Kinds of Liquid Supplements

There are several different kinds of liquid supplements designed for specific purposes. Consult with your doctor or dietitian before choosing one.

Polymeric

Standard versions of oral supplements are called polymeric because the carbohydrates, fats, and protein molecules are provided as complete undigested molecules. This is the way we would find them in food. Other products are designed to help with impaired digestion.

Semi-elemental

In semi-elemental products, the protein has been broken down (hydrolyzed) into smaller molecules. These smaller components of proteins are called peptides, and these can be made of two, three, or several amino acids joined together (amino acids are the most basic building block of protein).

Macronutrient Proportions

Most liquid supplements are designed to provide balanced nutrition, meaning that they provide the macronutrients (protein, carbohydrate, and fats) in healthy proportions: 50% to 55% of calories from carbohydrates, 15% to 20% of calories from protein, and less than 30% of calories from fat. Some specialized products may have a higher amount of protein, some may have different kinds of fat that may be more easily digested, and some may have added fiber.

Elemental

Another specialized type of supplement is called elemental because the protein is hydrolyzed into its most basic components (free amino acids). These supplements usually contain fats and carbohydrates in partially digested (simplest forms) as well.

These products are designed to be more easily absorbed when digestion is impaired. For this reason, they usually contain medium-chain triglycerides (MCT oil) as part of their fat content. MCTs do not require digestion and can be absorbed directly from the gut. The amount of fat in these specialized medical foods may also be reduced. The manufacturing companies are also starting to include more healthy fat sources, such as canola oil (to increase the amount of anti-inflammatory omega-3 fat) instead of corn oil (thus reducing the pro-inflammatory omega-6 fat content).

Modular

You may also wish to supplement just one specific nutrient. Medical products designed to do this are called modular supplements. Examples include Polycose (carbohydrate only), MCT oil (fat only), or protein powders. These can be added to many foods (easily added to liquids or moist foods). There are also calorie- or protein-boosting drinks that can be made with either cow's milk or soy beverage. Examples include Scandishake, which can provide close to 600 calories when made with 1 cup (250 mL) of whole milk, and Carnation Breakfast Anytime, which boosts calories and protein (but it does contain lactose).

Primary Therapy

For Crohn's disease affecting the small bowel, nutritional supplements can be used as primary therapy to treat the inflammation and thereby reduce symptoms. This is not the case for ulcerative colitis. When individuals drink only supplements (or receive supplements via a feeding tube), they often find their disease goes into remission and they can avoid steroid medications. This is especially important for children and adolescents who want to avoid the negative side effects of steroids, such as delayed growth. Polymeric, semi-elemental, or elemental supplements all provide a beneficial effect.

Different theories have been proposed to account for the effectiveness of these supplements in some patients. The sterile properties of the supplements, the beneficial effects of specific types of fat, and the beneficial effect of simply improving overall nutritional status, with a consequent improvement in immunity, may account for the effectiveness of supplements.

Full Requirements
Most liquid supplements have vitamins, minerals, and trace elements added. In order to meet the full requirements for these, a specific volume must be consumed. For an average person, you might need to drink four or five units (cans, boxes, tetra paks, or packages dissolved in water) every day in order to meet your needs.

Tips for Taking Supplements

- Discuss your supplements with your pharmacist because they are experts.
- Take fiber supplements separately because fiber may bind to some nutrients, thus interfering with their absorption.
- If supplementing fat-soluble vitamins, take with a meal because they require some fat to be better absorbed.
- If you require calcium supplements, take them separately from multivitamins because the iron in the multivitamin interferes with calcium absorption.
- Take medications cold (keep the container on ice) to ease swallowing.
- Mix supplements in water, cover, and sip with a straw to avoid the medicine odor.
- Flavor nutrition drinks with vanilla, mint, or banana extracts or flavor packets.
- Include in a milkshake or smoothie recipe.
- Substitute nutrition drinks for milk in baking recipes.

Low-Fiber Diets

Insoluble and Soluble Fiber

Both insoluble and soluble fiber are good for you, but if you are looking to reduce bowel movement frequency and thicken stool consistency, then you will probably want to increase your intake of soluble fiber. Likewise, to avoid increasing the frequency of bowel movements (such as during a disease flare), limit sources of insoluble fiber.

Dietitians and physicians usually recommend increasing fiber in your diet for overall good health. Fiber is important for weight management. Fiber may help manage blood sugar in diabetes, it may help manage diverticulosis, it may help reduce cholesterol, and it may help protect against some kinds of cancers. While eating fiber, you feel full sooner and may eat less. Despite these clear health benefits, your doctor or dietitian may ask you to limit fiber in your diet because you have IBD. The priority when you have an IBD flare is to recover, return to better health, and have improved quality of life. This may require adjusting or reducing your fiber intake.

In clinical practice, a low-residue diet limits foods that increase the amount of undigested food matter and the amount of stool produced. The definition of low residue is not well supported by evidence, and as such, clinicians now refer to a low-fiber diet. Low-fiber diets allow soluble fiber, but limit insoluble fiber and foods that could potentially contribute to food-related obstructions.

This fiber-restricted diet is intended only to be a short-term diet to help you feel more comfortable by decreasing gastrointestinal intolerance symptoms from a flare or from a change in the normal anatomy after surgery. This is not a fiber-free diet; rather, there is a compromise by allowing soluble fiber until you can comfortably include sources of insoluble fibre in your diet again. The goal is for you to return to a regular diet once your disease and symptoms have improved. In the meantime, be sure to plan meals in advance so that you can find acceptable alternatives and have them available to you when you are hungry.

Long-Term Low-Fiber Diet

There are times when a low-fiber diet needs to be followed over a longer period of time. Such is the case when you have narrowing of the bowel due to scar tissue or stricturing of the intestine in Crohn's disease. When there is narrowing, the bowels must push hard to pass undigested food matter through the narrowed area. This causes cramping, pain, and, in some cases, abdominal bloating and nausea.

Similar situations of bowel narrowing occur with inflammation from active Crohn's disease and bowel-wall swelling following surgery. This is usually temporary because the swelling decreases with treatment or time and the size of the opening of the bowel returns to normal. Unfortunately, scar tissue remains despite treatment with medication. In that case, the narrowing is permanent, unless it is surgically removed or corrected.

Cocktail Caution

Beware of so-called juice cocktails, because they only contain a small amount of natural fruit juice, while the rest is water with large amounts of sugar in the form of high-fructose corn syrup, dextrose, or sugar/glucose-fructose. Look for the label "100% fruit juice" or "100% juice blends." Natural juice provides more vitamins, minerals, trace elements, and natural antioxidants than juice cocktails.

Long-term compliance with a low-fiber diet brings unique challenges for ensuring that vitamins, minerals, and trace elements are adequate, considering the many restrictions to the fruits and vegetables food group. The key is to rely on fruits and vegetables that are canned, well cooked, squeezed into juices, or blenderized and strained. Sometimes a multivitamin and mineral supplement is needed, and these are now available for adults in chewable and "gummy" forms.

Fiber Fortification

To include more soluble fiber in your diet, try adding oat bran to moist foods, such as yogurt, pudding, sauces, and soups, as well as in baked goods (muffins or cookies) and cereal. You can even sprinkle oat bran onto your oatmeal! Try adding chickpeas or lentils to a casserole, or include kidney beans in a stew. You can substitute applesauce for oil in a muffin recipe (also lower fat!). Add barley to soup, or make split pea soup. Slice bananas into Jell-O or yogurt for dessert.

Fiber Sources

Insoluble Fiber	Soluble Fiber
• Skins of fruits and vegetables (e.g., skins of peppers, eggplant, tomato, corn, apple) • Seeds of fruits and vegetables (kiwi, oranges, eggplant, field cucumbers, tomato) • Membranes of fruits and vegetables (sections of oranges, grapefruit) • Whole wheat and whole-grain breads and cereals • Brown or wild rice • White whole wheat flour (contains the bran and germ and thus the same fiber as whole wheat but looks like refined flour)	• Oat products: oatmeal and oat bran (breads, muffins, cookies, hot or cold cereals) • Barley • Tapioca • Psyllium fiber (powder, biscuit, or capsule, including Metamucil, Prodiem, or generic house brands) • Methylcellulose (Citrucel) • Pectin • Banana flakes • Pulp of fruits (flesh of orange, applesauce, grapefruit, banana) • Vegetables (okra) • Legumes (chickpeas, kidney beans, lentils with outer skin peeled)

Food Label Caution

It is important to read labels when choosing products for fiber content. For example, if a food product lists bran as a component, it most likely is wheat bran, a source of insoluble fiber; however, if the product specifies "oat" in front of bran, as in "oat bran," it is a source of soluble fiber.

Kellogg's All-Bran Buds cereal with psyllium, for example, advertises one of the highest sources of fiber per serving. The label also lists "psyllium seed husk," which would lead one to think the cereal is a high source of psyllium and thus soluble fiber. Soluble fiber is good, right? The problem is that while each serving packs 3 g of soluble fiber, it also packs a whopping 9.7 g of insoluble fiber. If you read the ingredient list, wheat bran is the first listed ingredient, meaning that it constitutes the largest proportion of ingredients in the product. As a source of insoluble fiber, wheat bran will promote the opposite effect that you are looking for from the small soluble fiber content!

High-Stool-Output Management Diets

Sometimes modifying fiber isn't enough to slow down bowel movements. This can be the case during a flare or following multiple bowel resections if you have a high-output stoma or a pelvic pouch for ulcerative colitis. It is then appropriate to try some other diet strategies, provided you are receiving appropriate medical treatment for your condition.

There are many diet strategies that can be explored to help slow stool frequency and increase stool consistency. When making changes, try only one strategy at a time and for a few days. This way, if there is any benefit, you know what diet change is responsible. Conversely, you may find that you experience no positive effect, and you can then resume your usual intake and try other tips that might be helpful. Be sure to consult with your doctor or dietitians while trying these strategies.

Dietary Strategies to Slow High Stool Output

Modification	Explanation and Examples
• Increase soluble fiber	• Some people experience the most benefit from including soluble fiber at mealtime (not in between meals).
• Include foods known to thicken stool	• Cheese and cheesecake, smooth nut butters (peanut butter, almond butter, cashew butter), pretzels, potato chips, white rice (especially sticky rice like Arborio), tapioca, unleavened bread products (matzo and water crackers), gelatin-containing foods (Jell-O and marshmallows).
• Restrict dairy lactose	• If you reduce or eliminate dairy lactose, be sure to eat alternative calcium sources. • Try commercial lactase enzyme products.
• Reduce fat	• For extensive ileal Crohn's disease or ileal resection of more than 3 feet (1 m). This loss of bowel disrupts absorption of fat, and there is a greater loss of bile salts (normally reabsorbed in the ileum). • Try supplementing with MCT oil (available in specialty food shops), which is easily added to soups, beverages, salad dressings.
• Reduce simple sugars	• Sweets (jams, jellies, honey, maple syrup) and sweetened beverages (ice tea, fruit drinks, pop, soda, sports drinks, chocolate milk). • Dilute concentrated sugar sources, such as fruit juices, and sip slowly.
• Reduce fructose	• A monosaccharide found naturally in fruits, but also a component of high-fructose corn syrup added to fruit drinks, soft drinks, baked goods, such as cookies. • Can cause an osmotic diarrhea at higher intakes (tolerance level is different for different people). • Fermented in colon by bacteria, thus contributing to gas.
• Reduce sugar alcohols	• Nutritive sweeteners that have about half the calories of regular sugar. Examples include sorbitol, mannitol, xylitol, and hydrogenated starch hydrolysates. • Found in hard candies, gum, mints, jams, and jellies. • Poorly absorbed and fermented in colon, contributing to gas, cramping, bloating, and diarrhea.
• Try gas-reducing strategies	• Gas is produced when fiber and residue from complex carbohydrates reach the colon. • Plan regular snacks between meals to reduce gas production (keep canned fruit with peel-back lids, granola bars, or individually wrapped oat bran cookies in your car's glove compartment or in a desk drawer at work.)

Modification	Explanation and Examples
• Try gas-reducing strategies (continued)	• If taking carbonated beverages, pour into a glass first and let stand for 10–15 minutes to reduce the carbonation. • Try commercial enzyme products (e.g., Beano, Phazyme), which pre-digest fiber and residue without forming gas. • Avoid smoking, chewing gum, using straws. • Chew foods well.
• Reduce caffeine and eliminate guarana	• Caffeine sources include coffee, tea (including green tea), hot chocolate, soft drinks (including dark colas and Mountain Dew). • Guarana comes from a shrub in the rainforest (seeds from its fruit are crushed, and these contain caffeine and other xanthines that stimulate bowel peristalsis). Examples of drinks with guarana include some varieties of beer and energy drinks (Red Bull, XTC, GURU, Dark Dog, SoBe Adrenaline Rush). Avoid beer with added caffeine.
• Reduce alcohol	• Beer, drinks mixed with carbonated beverages, and red wine are particularly troublesome.
• Modify spices and seasonings	• Don't need to be eliminated. • Use ground pepper instead of whole peppercorns, mild curry instead of hot. • Important for keeping food flavorful and interesting.
• Adjust meal sizes and timing	• Eat 3 smaller meals, snacks in between. • Aim for 5–6 smaller meals per day. • Eat dinner early in the evening. Make lunch the main meal.
• Separate solids from liquids	• Consume solid food (e.g., a sandwich) and wait 30–45 minutes before consuming beverage. • Small sips of fluid with solid food is okay.
• Delay gastric emptying (provided that ileal brake mechanism is intact)	• Ileal brake is a feedback mechanism that helps to slow transit time of food through the bowel by regulating how quickly the stomach empties. • Ensure fat and protein are components of each meal. • Focus on complex carbohydrates and inclusion of soluble fiber.

Antidiarrheal Medications

Antidiarrheal medications are another strategy that can provide some relief and help you regain some quality of life. For instance, if you are not able to sleep throughout the night due to high stool outputs, medication can be used temporarily to reduce frequency so you can sleep a little longer. Sleeping better may in turn help you to cope better. Examples of medications that can help to slow high stool outputs are Imodium, Lomotil, Questran, and codeine phosphate.

Fluid Diet Challenges

The challenge with fluid diets is getting enough nutrition, because most fluids aren't balanced with adequate vitamins, minerals, protein, and other essential nutrients.

Fluid Diets

For a short time following surgery, while experiencing obstructive symptoms, or during a flare, you may need to follow a fluid diet to relieve your symptoms by eliminating most indigestible food matter (also called residue). You might also be asked to follow a liquid-only diet if you have a fistula.

Even though you don't have much of an appetite under these conditions, you may find that you are able to drink fluids. However, while on a fluid diet, it may be difficult to consume enough calories to maintain your weight.

Clear Fluid Diets

Unfortunately, clear fluids are not a balanced source of nutrition, and are especially lacking in calories and protein. A clear fluid diet should generally be limited to no longer than several days. On this diet, you can easily develop taste fatigue and boredom with the lack of variety, texture, smell, and taste.

Examples of clear fluids are strained vegetable or meat broths, tea, coffee, clear popsicles, Jell-O, clear juices or cocktails, such as apple or cranberry, fruit punch and other sweetened drinks, soda pop, and specially prepared nutritional products, such as Resource Fruit Beverage. Clear fluids flavored or sweetened with strained lemon juice, honey, sugar, or artificial sweeteners are considered to be fine.

Full Fluid Diets

Slightly more nutritious is the full fluid diet because of the addition of some dairy products or alternatives, such as soy milk for lactose intolerant individuals or vegans (when all animal products are avoided). Still, it is difficult to meet protein requirements on the full fluid diet.

Examples of full fluids are milk, cream, soy milk, strained hot cereals (oatmeal, cream of wheat), puddings, custard, ice cream, sorbet, gelato, strained cream soups, fruit juices, vegetable juice, and nutritional products that are "creamier" in texture (for example, Ensure, Boost, Resource, and pharmacy house brands).

Maintaining Hydration and Electrolyte Balance

The more fluid you lose in your stool, the more likely you are to experience dehydration. If you have had your colon removed (where fluid and electrolytes are primarily absorbed), your small intestine will partially adapt to take over this function, but this takes time, and the stool will become pasty at best. When passing frequent liquid stool, be sure that you are getting adequate fluids and replacing electrolytes.

Best Fluids

Fluids that are best absorbed match the concentration, or osmolality, of your body fluids. This allows for the best absorption or transfer of fluid across the cell membranes in your intestine. An example of a good replacement fluid would be Gastrolyte for adults or Pedialyte for children. Milk, juices, and sports drinks (for example, Gatorade) are not absorbed as well due to their higher sugar content and consequent higher osmolality (a measure of the concentration of molecules dissolved in water).

Water may be better absorbed than the sugary drinks, such as juices. When there is a high sugar concentration in a fluid, drinking it results in fluid shifting into the intestine from the tissues, instead of out of the intestine into the tissues and the bloodstream, thereby leading to more watery stool. You can try diluting concentrated sugar sources, such as juices and sports drinks, and sip them slowly to avoid the problem of increased diarrhea. There also are some reduced sugar sports drinks available; these are sweetened with artificial sweeteners instead of sugar.

Also beware of fluids that are known to increase urine production and loss of water from the body — otherwise known as a diuretic effect. Examples of these fluids include caffeinated beverages and alcohol. There is even a combination of these two diuretics — a new kind of beer on the market that has added caffeine. Caffeinated beverages include dark colas (Coke, Pepsi, house-brand colas, root beer) and clear soft drinks (Mountain Dew), coffee, tea (including green tea), chocolate, and hot chocolate. Some medications, such as over-the-counter cold and flu remedies, also contain caffeine.

> **Dehydration Symptoms**
>
> Symptoms of dehydration and electrolyte loss include fatigue, feeling light-headed or faint, increased thirst, dry mouth, stomach cramps, and decreased urine output, to name a few. A rapid loss in weight from day to day is another indicator of dehydration.

Sodium and Potassium Sources

Mineral	Source
Sodium	• Canned soups and vegetables • Tomato sauce • Bullion cubes • Snack foods (e.g., pretzels, salted crackers, potato chips, salted popcorn, corn chips) • Fast foods • Processed foods (e.g., processed cheese, processed and smoked meats) • Canned fish (e.g., tuna, salmon, sardines, anchovies) and dried fish (e.g., dried cod or herring) • Canned legumes • Ready-to-eat cereals (e.g., instant oatmeal) • Sauces and condiments (e.g., soy, Worcestershire, and barbecue sauces, salad dressings, ketchup, relish, pickles) • Table salt
Potassium	• Potatoes • Oranges • Nectarines • Mangoes • Bananas • Tomato products (soup, sauce, paste) • Avocado • Melon (cantaloupe, honeydew, watermelon) • Apricots • Juices (orange, carrot, tomato, vegetable, passion fruit) • Coconut water • Asparagus • Legumes (chickpeas, lentils, split peas, kidney beans, soybeans) • Beets • Parsnips • Sweet potato/yam • Pumpkin • Okra • Barley • Salt substitute • Smooth nut butters • Brown sugar • Molasses • Maple syrup • Strong tea and coffee • Chocolate

Electrolytes

Sodium and potassium are two electrolytes critical for regulation and balance of body fluids. They can be found in many foods in small amounts, but it is best to target higher sources on a regular basis if there is any concern with dehydration risk.

Food Fears

If you've lived for a long time with an intestinal stricture and diet restrictions, it can be daunting to try new foods again after surgery has removed the stricture. If you have ever experienced a bowel obstruction as a result of the food you have eaten, the motivation to avoid pain and just "stay away" from suspicious or questionable foods is quite strong. It is normal to feel apprehensive about liberalizing your diet again, but slowly, with time, you will feel more comfortable with the function of your gut's new anatomy and digestion. It is important to chew food slowly and thoroughly, to eat small portion sizes, and to retry one new food at a time.

One goal of diet modifications is to facilitate an improved relationship with food and eating. All strategies that potentially restrict the types and varieties of foods should be reassessed periodically so they can be adjusted and a regular diet can be resumed.

Sometimes, despite your best efforts, diet modifications just do not have the desired effect. This could mean that your disease is active and requires medical therapy.

Nutrition Support

If there is risk of developing malnutrition or progression of malnutrition, sometimes a more intensive and defined form of nutrition, called nutrition support, is required. There are two types of nutrition support, total enteral nutrition (tube feeding) and total parenteral nutrition (intravenous feeding).

Tube Feeding

By itself, total enteral nutrition (TEN) can reduce the amount of inflammation in the intestine and thereby avoid the need for medications, such as steroids, that may have numerous undesirable side effects. It also has the added benefit of enhancing growth.

A relatively soft, small tube is passed through the nose and through the esophagus, ending up in the stomach or upper part of the small intestine. Tube feeding can be delivered by using gravity drip or a pump to deliver a precise volume per hour. Tube feeding does not preclude taking other fluids by mouth, so you can continue to drink even while you have the tube inserted.

Children often learn how to place this tube themselves. They insert the tube every evening before going to bed, administer the feeds overnight while they sleep, and take the tube out in the morning before going about their usual activities during the day.

The procedure should be supervised by your health-care team to ensure that possible side effects of tube feeding (bloating, cramping, diarrhea) are monitored and properly addressed. There is also a cost associated with tube feeding, which is not always covered by governments or third parties, such as insurance companies.

TEN

In total enteral nutrition, nutritional supplements are delivered via a feeding tube when you are just not able to consume enough by mouth. This method of nutrition support is particularly helpful in children with certain forms of IBD, particularly Crohn's disease of the small intestine.

Intravenous Nutrition

Total parenteral nutrition (TPN) is a specialized form of nutrition delivered via an intravenous line. A PICC (peripherally inserted central catheter) line is an example of a type of line that is commonly placed to deliver the concentrated nutrients to a large blood vessel, which rapidly dilutes the solution. In this kind of nutrition support, the gut can rest because no absorption is required while nutrients are delivered directly into the bloodstream.

TPN may be required before surgery if you are very ill and cannot consume enough nutrition by mouth or by tube feeding. Sometimes after surgery the bowel is slow to work; TPN can be provided until this resolves and you are eating well again. With multiple surgeries for Crohn's disease, some individuals don't have enough intestines left to absorb adequate nutrients and maintain stable weight, fluid balance, and electrolyte balance. These people may need TPN permanently, in which case there are home TPN programs available in many communities to prescribe and monitor the administration of TPN.

TPN

In total parenteral nutrition, nutrients in a solution are administered directly into a person's vein by means of an intravenous line.

This may seem like a perfect solution to avoid the discomfort of gastrointestinal intolerance symptoms from eating. Besides the high cost, there are, however, risks that need to be taken into account before making a decision to use TPN. These include a higher risk of infection, blood clots (deep vein thrombosis), and metabolic intolerance. Because this is an artificial way to provide nutrition, your body often has difficulty processing the nutrients, and you could develop problems with your liver or gallbladder or abnormalities of cholesterol, triglycerides, and sugar levels in the blood as a result. Some people do not feel hungry while on TPN because the intravenous solution is giving them enough calories, but they sometimes do psychologically miss eating food and want to eat.

A specialized nutrition support team can help to avoid these complications while monitoring and adjusting the TPN to account for blood values that are unstable or abnormal.

Current Nutrition Research

Many people are hopeful that nutrition may play a role not only in treating but also in preventing IBD. There are several areas of research that hold this promise.

Synbiotics

"Synbiotics" refers to both prebiotics and probiotics, which contribute to maintaining the health of the intestinal bacteria and keep a sufficient number of "good" bacteria in the intestine.

Bacteria in the intestinal tract are important factors in maintaining an appropriate balance within the body's immune system. The inflammatory response is actually a natural protective mechanism, but can be damaging if it is overactive or uncontrolled. It is thought that some of the "good" bacteria normally present in the intestine contribute to maintaining the appropriate balance of the immune response.

There are food sources of both prebiotics and probiotics, but how much and how often you should eat these foods to experience benefits is not known.

Prebiotics

Prebiotics are non-digestible carbohydrates that are fermented by colonic bacteria. The process of fermentation provides energy for the growth of "good" bacteria, which, in turn, produce short-chain fatty acids, which are a fuel source for the cells lining the large intestine. Prebiotics also promote water and electrolyte reabsorption.

Prebiotics known as fructo-oligosaccharides (FOS) can be found in everyday foods, such as onions, bananas, tomatoes, honey, garlic, barley, and wheat. Some nutrition companies are adding these prebiotics to their food supplement drinks and puddings.

More recently, food companies have been adding a prebiotic named inulin (a soluble fiber processed from chicory root) to dairy products, chocolate, and beverages. Interestingly, most soluble fibers, including psyllium fiber, are considered prebiotics.

Probiotics

Probiotics are any number of different "good" live bacteria that are administered by mouth, in a capsule or in a drink or food, and confer a health benefit. The bacteria then establish themselves and grow within the intestine, a process called colonization. They are thought to provide immune system balance by down-regulating inflammation.

Live bacteria are most easily found in yogurts, where active bacterial cultures have been added. Unfortunately, there is no standardization regarding the bacterial strains or amount of bacterial colony forming units (CFUs) added. Similarly, the amount of remaining live bacteria when you consume the product will be affected by the processing, transport, and storage conditions. Live bacteria need to be kept in a refrigerated environment. Probiotics must also arrive alive in the gut, so they must be acid- and bile-resistant.

Examples of probiotics include *Lactobacillus acidophilus* and bifidobacterium. When buying yogurt, look for those that "contain" active cultures as compared with those that are "made with" active cultures to be sure you're getting as much of the live bacteria as possible. It is important to know the strain of bacteria because not all strains in a given group have the same benefit.

Immunonutrition (Omega-3 Fatty Acids)

This rapidly expanding area of nutrition is of interest wherever there is an inflammatory component to disease (for example, arthritis, cardiovascular disease, IBD). Immunonutrition involves modulating the inflammatory response through diet.

Limits

As with all fermentable foods, be sure to limit your intake of prebiotics to only a few grams a day in order to avoid gas and cramping. When foods are fermented by bacteria in the intestine, gas is produced as a normal by-product. Although not abnormal, gas may be uncomfortable or, in some situations, socially unacceptable.

Pouchitis Prevention

VSL#3 is a pharmaceutical probiotic preparation containing eight different bacterial strains and three billion viable bacteria per gram that has shown promising results for preventing recurrent pouchitis (an inflammation of the pelvic pouch created from the end of small bowel when the colon is removed due to ulcerative colitis).

The type of fat we eat is directly related to the fat that makes up our cells, which influences a cell's ability to produce eicosanoids and cytokines. These are hormone-like compounds that affect the body's immune response to injury and infection. By eating more anti-inflammatory fats, we can directly influence production of these anti-inflammatory mediators.

There are a few different kinds of dietary fats, including trans fats, saturated fats, monounsaturated fats, and polyunsaturated fats (PUFAs), including the essential omega-3 and omage-6 PUFAs. "Essential" means that our body cannot make those fatty acids and we can only get them through our diet. Two important omega-3 fatty acids are eicosapentaenoic acid (EPA) and docosahexaenoic acid (DHA). You will get these from fish and seafood. Another omage-3 fatty acid is alpha linolenic acid (ALA), and you get this from plant-based foods.

Essential Fatty Acids (Omega-3 and Omega-6) Sources

Omega-6	Omega-3
Vegetable oils • Corn oil • Sunflower oil • Safflower oil • Cottonseed oil (Can also be found in processed foods and commercial baked goods)	**Oils** • Canola oil • Walnut oil • Flaxseed oil • Fish oil • Ground flaxseed (add in baked goods, add to moist foods like yogurt, applesauce, sauces) • Hemp seeds • Chia seeds (salba seeds) • Dark green leafy vegetables • Soybeans • Cold water fatty fish: salmon, tuna, trout, mackerel, anchovy, sardines, sturgeon, bluefish, mullet, herring (menhaden) • Functional foods: omega-3 eggs, DHA milk, soy beverages, cheese, yogurt, margarine, organic grain cereals (some of these foods contain only marginally higher amounts)

Notes: Fish oil supplements are often made from fish skin and liver and may contain environmental contaminants. Check ingredient labels for more information. Consider omega-3 (DHA) supplements made from algae instead.

Functional foods are conventional foods (fish, for example) or those similar in appearance to a conventional food (omega-3 eggs, for example) that are part of a usual diet and that demonstrate a physiological health benefit.

Optimal Dose

The optimal amount of omega-3 in the diet has not been defined in IBD. In cardiovascular disease, the optimal intake has been defined as 1000 mg EPA plus DHA per day. For the general public, some recommendations in the medical literature suggest an intake of 400 to 500 mg per day as being optimal. While ALA is not as efficiently converted to EPA and DHA in the body, it is still recommended (National Academy of Sciences) that women need 1100 mg and men 1600 mg per day.

To put this in perspective, one omega-3 egg has roughly 5 mg EPA and 75 mg DHA. Omega-3 milk has roughly 15 mg DHA per cup (250 mL). Some of these products have added costs, so be sure to read the label to determine whether the additional omega-3 is significant enough to add to your daily totals.

Marine sources of omega-3 are the best sources of EPA and DHA, the forms most easily used by the body. ALA from plant sources is only partially converted by the body to EPA and DHA. Still, it is considered worthwhile to include plant sources of omega-3 along with marine sources because this can improve the balance of omega-3 to omega-6 fatty acids in the diet. It is also thought that ALA may help the body's metabolism of blood sugar.

Antioxidants

The area of antioxidants and IBD looks promising, but studies are still at a biochemical level and cannot yet be translated to specific recommendations for people. Antioxidants include vitamin E, vitamin C, carotenoids, glutathione, and selenium.

Microparticles

There is also a so-called low-microparticle diet being studied for relief of symptoms in Crohn's disease. This diet involves avoiding inert inorganic non-nutrient microparticles. These include natural contaminants, such as soil and dust, as well as food additives, such as aluminosilicates and titanium dioxide used as brightening agents or anti-caking agents. The diet also focuses on avoiding processed foods, such as processed meats and processed cheese, or anything that could have soil residue. There is not yet strong evidence to support its use in clinical practice.

Trophic Factors

Trophic (growth or anabolic) factors, such as glutamine, have also generated interest. Glutamine is an amino acid (building block of protein) that the body can make on its own. During times of stress, it is considered "conditionally essential" because the body cannot produce enough for the demand. Because it is a fuel source for intestinal mucosa and immune cells, glutamine has been proposed to help with Crohn's disease and short bowel syndrome, but research has not demonstrated any benefit to date. There are limited human studies, and stability is an issue with some supplement forms of glutamine.

Glucagon is another protein that looks promising for the treatment of short bowel syndrome, as it helps to stimulate improved intestinal function.

Diet Counseling

While there is no standard diet for IBD, diet modifications can help with symptom management. Diet restrictions are usually temporary during times of disease activity or post-operative recovery periods.

Any diet modifications should be discussed with your doctor or dietitian. Changes to usual food choices need to be practical and realistic,while taking into consideration individual choices for reasons of religion, culture, ethnicity, beliefs, personal food preferences, tolerances, allergies, phobias, lifestyle, employment, sports, and financial considerations. This is why diet modifications aren't just about changing something like fiber in your diet; they are individualized recommendations that work for you as an individual living with IBD.

CHAPTER 6

Psychological Support for Managing IBD

Dr. Bob Maunder and Dr. A. Hillary Steinhart

CASE STUDIES Susan and Jerome

Susan is 22, in her fourth year of university. She was diagnosed with ulcerative colitis at the age of 17. She is frustrated with the course of her disease. Diarrhea, fatigue, and the medication she takes all seem to interfere with her concentration at school. She has decided that she wants to look into pelvic pouch surgery, but doesn't know whether she should take more time off school for the operation or try to schedule it in the summer break. "I never know whether I am pushing myself too hard," she tells her doctor, "or if I just need to keep trying to live a normal life at a normal pace."

Jerome, 42, teaches at a high school and has been living with Crohn's disease for 20 years. Given the time constraints of his job, he used to find it difficult to get through the day without interruption or fear of embarrassment. In recent years, he has found strategies to cope with these pressures. "I don't have any choice about what time I start my day," he explains. "Mornings are usually tricky for me because I'm likely to have to go to the bathroom a few times before 9:00. It used to be more of a stress, but now I eat a smaller breakfast and drive to work instead of taking the bus, so I'm less likely to have to go really badly, and if I do I can stop at a public washroom. I know where all of the washrooms are on my route to work!"

Psychological Concerns

Once considered by some health-care professionals as psychosomatic illnesses, we now know that Crohn's disease and ulcerative colitis are not caused by personality or other psycho-logical factors. Although we have learned a great deal about the experience of living with inflammatory bowel disease, there is much that we don't yet understand about the relationship between mind and body. One thing is certain: if you have inflammatory bowel disease, you should pay attention to what is happening to you emotionally during the course of your illness and how the illness affects your life and your relationships.

The range of psychological issues relevant to IBD is large. Some challenges affect almost everybody with IBD to some extent. These include finding ways to live with the uncertainty inherent in the disease. Other common challenges are tolerating physical symptoms, such as fatigue and pain, and dealing with the ways the disease affects relationships, ranging from concerns about the way that embarrassment may affect day-to-day relationships to concerns about burdening friends and family at times when you need to depend on them. Some challenges may not affect all people with IBD but require extra attention, such as the role of stress in triggering a flare of inflammation, or complications leading to depression.

Developing strategies for relieving and preventing stress and depression is important for managing IBD and improving your quality of life. The fundamental strategy is to know yourself. Think about your experience with health problems and with other challenges in your life. What have you done that has helped in the past? What has been less successful? Who in your life has been most supportive? Where can you turn for support? We'll help you answer these questions.

Quality of Life

While psychological factors do not cause your disease and while psychological changes will not cure it, your mental attitude and the way that you understand your illness can contribute significantly to your quality of life. Seek psychological support from health-care professionals, family members, and friends to manage your condition.

Psychological Factors in IBD Management

Besides coping with the pain and fatigue your disease may be causing, there are other psychological factors that may cause considerable discomfort. In more serious cases, these factors may lead to chronic stress and depression.

Uncertainty: How can I predict the course of my disease hour to hour, day to day, and month to month? When will the next flare occur?

Embarrassment: How do I talk about this disease with family, friends, and acquaintances when bowel symptoms are not usually part of polite conversation?

Anxiety: How do I find or keep a romantic partner when I have a bowel disease?

Worry: What physical and mental abilities will be affected by the disease? Will I be able to maintain my family, social, work, and educational responsibilities?

Adjustment: What adjustments will I need to make to my plans for the future?

Dependence: Are my loved ones going to get tired of me if I depend on them too much?

Guilt: Am I trying hard enough?

Doubt: Is it okay to ask for help?

Q **What is the role of stress in IBD?**

A Scientific research into the role of stress in triggering flares of illness in patients with Crohn's disease or ulcerative colitis is about evenly split between studies that find a link and studies that find no link between stress and these diseases. These studies have shown the following evidence, however:

- Personality has no impact on whether or not a person develops IBD.
- Life stresses probably have no impact on whether or not a person develops IBD.
- Life stress may be one of the factors that can trigger a flare of disease when disease has been inactive, but this is probably only true for some people with IBD.

Stress

While stress does not cause Crohn's disease or ulcerative colitis, these conditions do cause stress for patients and their families. Coping with the pain and fatigue, as well as complicated decisions about treatment, clearly can be stressful, but some of the strongest sources of stress for people with IBD are less obvious.

Patient perception of the role of stress is also split. About 1 in 3 people with IBD believe that stress or psychological factors had something to do with getting the illness in the first place. About 3 in 4 people believe that stress affects the course of their disease.

In determining whether stress is a factor in your IBD, try to distinguish between experiencing common gut symptoms and active inflammation (a flare of disease). An increase in symptoms does not always mean that the intestine is inflamed. You can experience increased fatigue, pain, or diarrhea for many reasons other than IBD. In fact, these symptoms of an irritable bowel are quite common in IBD even when there is no active inflammation. There is some evidence that once a person's bowel has been affected by repeated occurrences of inflammation and healing, it is more likely to respond to stress with diarrhea and pain, even if a flare of inflammation doesn't occur.

Until there is better evidence upon which to base decisions, the best policy seems to be to know yourself and trust your experience. If you believe from your own experience with IBD that the stresses in your life (or the way that you react to them) have an impact on your symptoms, then it makes sense to try to modify the ways that you respond to stress. If your experience is that your disease course doesn't seem to depend on what is happening in your life, then you are probably right.

Maintaining Your Resilience to Stress

- Try to maintain a stable, predictable pattern of sleep, healthy diet, and moderate exercise. Although the symptoms of IBD may make it challenging to eat, exercise, and sleep, these can be powerful tools to maximize your health. It is very hard to manage stress effectively when you are sleep-deprived or malnourished.
- Try to identify and fix problems as they occur. The trick to this strategy is that it is usually the constructive effort to try to solve a problem that reduces stress, rather than the solution itself. Don't focus single-mindedly on the outcome of your efforts.
- Try to accept and tolerate the problems that can't be fixed. Whether or not you are religious, remember the Serenity Prayer: **God grant me the serenity to accept the things I cannot change, the courage to change the things I can, and the wisdom to know the difference.**
- Keep a sense of humor.
- Engage with life. Be an active part of your family, your circle of friends, and your community.
- Attend to your spiritual needs.
- Learn and use relaxation techniques or meditation.
- Take time for leisure.
- Avoid caffeine.

Depression

Depression is a very common illness. It would be surprising if you did not know someone who has lived with depression, since approximately 1 in 5 women and 1 in 10 men will experience a major depression at some point in their life. Depression is different from normal sadness or discouragement because it has a wider range of effects on feeling, thinking, and physical function and because, if not treated, it usually persists for weeks or months.

People who live with chronic diseases, such as IBD, are at increased risk of experiencing depression. There are probably many reasons for the increased risk. The losses and frustrations that come with living with a disease; the biological effects of inflammation (since many of the body's chemicals that increase immunity and inflammation also have effects on the brain); and the effects of medications, such as prednisone, may all contribute to depression.

Recognizing the symptoms of depression when it occurs is very important, because depression usually responds well to

> ### Successful Treatments
>
> Fortunately, depression can be treated effectively. The most effective forms of treatment are antidepressant medications, certain modes of psychotherapy or counseling, or a combination of these. If you think you are depressed, you should talk to your doctor.

treatment. Some of these symptoms may be hard to interpret when you have ulcerative colitis or Crohn's disease. Most people experience one or two of these symptoms some of the time without being depressed. Some can be caused by physical illness without being depressed. However, if symptoms persist and seem out of proportion to your usual experience of illness, talk to your doctor about the possibility of depression.

Vicious Cycle

If it is not treated, depression adds substantially to the burden of illness. People with chronic disease who are also depressed tend to experience more pain, fatigue, and other symptoms. Depression makes it harder to keep up your motivation to see the doctor when IBD symptoms emerge and to stick to your treatment plan. If you are depressed, you are less likely to be able to work and you are less likely to be effective in all of your efforts to cope with IBD. The result is that depression and IBD can make each other worse in a vicious cycle.

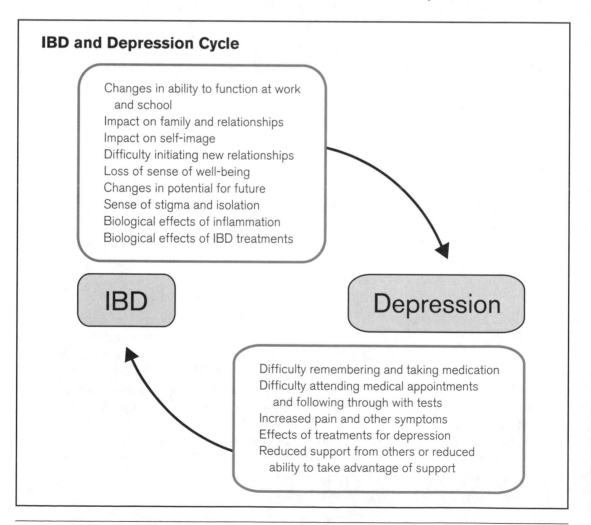

IBD and Depression Cycle

Changes in ability to function at work and school
Impact on family and relationships
Impact on self-image
Difficulty initiating new relationships
Loss of sense of well-being
Changes in potential for future
Sense of stigma and isolation
Biological effects of inflammation
Biological effects of IBD treatments

IBD

Depression

Difficulty remembering and taking medication
Difficulty attending medical appointments and following through with tests
Increased pain and other symptoms
Effects of treatments for depression
Reduced support from others or reduced ability to take advantage of support

Treating Depression

Depression can be effectively treated with antidepressant drugs or with certain forms of psychotherapy. Very often these forms of treatment are most effective if used together.

Drug Therapy

There are many effective antidepressant drugs available now. Your doctor can help you to choose the drug that is best suited to your situation.

Treating depression requires daily use of antidepressants for several months, often longer. However, depressive symptoms usually start to improve after taking an antidepressant for about 2 weeks, although it may take up to 12 weeks to feel the full benefit.

With modern antidepressant drugs, side effects (such as tremor, difficulty sleeping, or upset stomach) are usually not difficult to tolerate. Side effects are usually strongest shortly after starting a new medication or increasing the dose, and tend to settle down after a couple of weeks. Your doctor can help you to find a drug that is compatible with your IBD symptoms and its treatment.

Psychotherapy

Some forms of psychotherapy (talk therapy) are as effective as antidepressant drugs for treating moderately severe depression. Cognitive-behavioral therapy and interpersonal therapy, for example, have been found to be highly effective in many studies of depression. Other forms of psychotherapy may also be effective.

In cognitive-behavioral therapy, you learn to identify patterns of thought that tend to lead to depression or that tend to make depressive feelings worse. It is very common for people with depression to evaluate their experience in a way that leads to negative conclusions. Seeing things as black or white (all good or all bad), for example, means that many experiences and events are labeled as being bad, just because they aren't perfect. Many depressed people find that they pay close attention to negative or unhappy events and do not pay the same degree of attention to positive events, which tends to reinforce a pessimistic view. Patients work with their therapist to recognize their typical patterns of thought, to re-evaluate how accurate they are, and to develop alternative modes of thought. Typically cognitive-behavioral therapy occurs weekly for 3 or 4 months, sometimes longer.

In interpersonal therapy, patients work through, with their therapist, the feelings that are associated with an important life event linked to the current period of depression. Typical examples are grief over the death of a loved one, dealing with

---

Common Symptoms of Depression

- Lack of interest in things that are usually interesting to you
- Feeling excessively guilty or sad
- "Low" mood that doesn't improve when circumstances improve
- Feeling helpless about the present or hopeless about the future
- Low self-esteem or feelings of worthlessness
- Not participating in social activities even though you are physically well enough
- Thinking about suicide or being preoccupied with death
- Reduced appetite
- Reduced energy
- Poor concentration and memory
- Sleep disturbance

---

the mixed feelings of making a critical developmental transition (such as moving from living with family to living on your own), dealing with conflict in a partner relationship, or coping with social isolation. Interpersonal therapy also typically occurs weekly for 3 to 4 months, sometimes longer.

Coping Strategies

Much of what occurs in the course of living with IBD is not precisely under your control. Try to focus your attention on the things that you can control and use these to your advantage. Your own individual style of relating to yourself and to others may have a big influence on how you experience disease. So it is helpful to know your behavioral style and how it may affect your experience of IBD.

1. Know Your Interpersonal Style

One useful way of describing personal style is to look at how you prefer to relate to the people who are closest to you at times of stress. Do you look for the company of your partner or family members to talk things through and to feel supported? Do you depend on others to care for you when you are feeling overwhelmed? Do you find that you want to retreat from others and handle things alone?

People differ in the way they use close relationships to feel comfortable and secure at times of stress, and these differences have an impact on medical care. The impact of interpersonal style on medical care has received careful study in the last few years. Bear in mind that many things in addition to interpersonal style determine health outcomes.

Coping Strengths

People differ in their coping strengths, but, in general, the ways of coping that seem to be the most productive for most people are problem-solving, seeking emotional and practical support from others, looking for the positives in challenging situations, maintaining realistic expectations, and keeping a sense of humor. Less successful ways of coping, in general, include pretending that there isn't a problem (denial), avoiding any response, and acting out of anger.

Relationship Questionnaire

(adapted from Dr. Kim Bartholomew)

Look at these four basic interpersonal styles and see which one is the closest match to your style. Check the description that is closest to your relationship style.

Adaptable

It's easy for me to become emotionally close to others. I'm comfortable depending on them and having them depend on me. I don't worry about being alone or having others not accept me.

Support-seeking

I want to be completely emotionally intimate with others, but I often find that others are reluctant to get as close as I would like. I'm uncomfortable being without close relationships, but I sometimes worry that others don't value me as much as I value them.

Self-reliant

I'm comfortable without close emotional relationships. It's very important to me to feel independent and self-sufficient, and I prefer not to depend on others or have others depend on me.

Cautious

I'm uncomfortable getting close to others. I want emotionally close relationships, but I find it difficult to trust others completely or to depend on them. I worry that I will be hurt if I allow myself to become too close to others.

Adaptable Style

The adaptable style is usually associated with relative ease in using medical resources because people with this style tend to be comfortable with independence and with depending on others. Adaptable individuals are usually comfortable monitoring their situation independently and making their own health choices. They are also able turn to others for assistance when the situation demands.

Support-Seeking Style

People with the support-seeking style are more comfortable and may function more effectively when the people they count upon for support are near. People with a support-seeking style who have very supportive people in their life look and act very similar to people with an adaptable style. However, without good support from others, a person with a support-seeking style may be troubled by worry and negative feelings.

In general, the support-seeking style is associated with reporting more intense symptoms and a greater number of

Easy to Work With

Depending on how you measure things, about 30% to 60% of people have an adaptable interpersonal style. Health-care professionals usually report that it is easy to work with someone with an adaptable style, even if the medical situation is complicated.

symptoms (including ones that aren't typical for IBD or due to IBD). The support-seeking style is associated with more frequent visits to the doctor, and more tests. This may relate to a greater need for reassurance from others in order to feel comfortable. When IBD is active, the support-seeking style is associated with a higher risk of depression. Doctors of support-seeking patients find it easier to appreciate the significance of the changes in the course of IBD when they have known each other long enough for the doctor to recognize the patient's style of communication. Otherwise, there is a risk of overestimating the current level or severity of disease activity.

Self-Reliant Style

The self-reliant style is characterized by the lowest levels of symptom reporting. Visits to the doctor are infrequent. When it comes to one's health, a self-reliant interpersonal style may be a positive or a negative influence.

When managing diseases that require a great deal of collaboration between patients and health-care professionals, a self-reliant style can interfere, especially when patients do not disclose the whole picture of their current state or when a lack of collaboration is frustrating for the patient or the health-care provider. Doctors may need to schedule regular visits or tests rather than wait for a self-reliant patient to decide it is time to check in.

Cautious Style

The cautious style includes a push and pull when it comes to dealing with others, which can be tricky to balance in a medical setting. When a level of discomfort in managing things on one's own is combined with cautiousness about being willing to approach others or depend on them for help, a person with the cautious style may sometimes feel stuck.

These people are similar to self-reliant people in their relative underutilization of medical resources (preferring, for example, not to go to the doctor if it can be avoided), but are like people with a support-seeking style in their relatively greater experience of symptoms. If the situation calls for trying to overcome cautiousness, many people find it easiest to do this by finding one or two close confidants and relying on them to help with the challenges involved in being ill.

2. Know Your Information Gathering Style

A second way of understanding your behavioral style is to pay attention to how much information you like to have about your health. There is no right or wrong approach, but there

---

Self-Reliance Benefits and Risks

There is some evidence that self-reliant individuals have better health outcomes for some conditions. However, self-reliant individuals are prone to follow their own advice rather than seeking a professional opinion and may suffer silently with symptoms for longer than is reasonable.

Depression Risk

Like the support-seeking style, when IBD is active, people with a cautious style are at greater risk of becoming depressed.

---

are two main styles of collecting information, known to some psychologists as monitors or blunters. It helps to know your information gathering style because most of the time you will be most comfortable if you stick to your own style. It is also helpful to be aware of the ways in which these styles may lead to trouble if you overdo it.

Monitors

Some people feel most comfortable when they know everything. They prefer to monitor small changes in how they are feeling. They like to get opinions about what may be going on and what all the options are to treat their illness. Monitors often spend time on the Internet keeping up on the latest developments and researching all aspects of their medications. Monitors often find that it is comforting to gather more information (even if they don't end up acting on it).

Blunters

Other people only want information on a need-to-know basis. Blunters are often content to let their health-care providers recommend choices and don't want to know all of the details behind each choice. They may find that gathering extra information is anxiety-provoking rather than comforting. "Why should I hear about all of the things that might happen in the future? I'd rather just deal with things as they come up" is something that a blunter might say.

3. Know When Stress Is Beyond Your Comfort Zone

Often people respond to challenges that feel within their grasp through problem-solving and persistence, but respond to circumstances that are beyond their personal resources with emotional distress — feelings of grief, panic, or giving up. These are normal responses to extraordinary circumstances and shouldn't be interpreted as a sign of personal weakness or failure.

When stress feels like it is passing beyond your comfort zone, it is time to step back and reassess your options. Review the situation to see if the problem-solving strategies and helpful attitudes that usually work for you might work in this situation as well. Consider new ways of coping. For example, if you are a person who usually perseveres through trouble with a stiff upper lip, maybe now is a time to consider allowing yourself a breather and asking for help. In general, when stress crosses beyond the limits of your comfort zone, it is a good idea to consider allowing others to help.

Information Gathering Risks

The risk for monitors is that they will continue to gather information when it is no longer serving any useful purpose. For example, after you have gathered all of the information you need to make informed decisions, further exhaustive Internet searches of dubious sources of information can raise anxiety rather than awareness. The risk for blunters is that they may not gather enough information to be well-informed about their choices.

Taking Control of your IBD

Problem-Solving Strategies
- Get information
- Weigh your options
- Choose your best course
- Re-evaluate

Helpful Attitudes
- Look for the positives in challenging situations
- Maintain realistic expectations
- Keep a sense of humor

Many of these general rules depend on context, of course. The difference between having a sense of humor about events that aren't very funny and denying the reality of your situation is only a matter of degree. Similarly, the difference between the healthy assertiveness of insisting on your rights as a health consumer versus angry hostility toward those who want to help is a difference that may be in the eye of the beholder.

4. Turn to Others

Often, at times of crisis, it is very helpful to call upon the support of others, including family and friends who can offer practical support and can "be there for you" emotionally as good listeners. Moral support and practical help are usually more valuable than free advice. Professionals may be able to offer treatment and management options that have not been considered, which may also help to move illness challenges back into the realm where they feel manageable again.

Recognizing Obstacles

You have many resources to draw upon to help you with the challenges of illness, including your family and friends, health-care professionals, peer support groups, and your community. Sometimes you may want to turn to others, but you experience obstacles. Pay attention to these obstacles to see what is within your control. If you feel that you cannot turn to others for support, ask yourself why. Why are you reluctant to depend on someone else? Do you feel guilty burdening them? Were you disappointed in how they responded in the past? Many people face challenges of this kind, especially with partners, close friends, and family. You probably need to identify the type of obstacle you are experiencing before you can overcome it.

Improving Communication

Clear communication is often your most powerful tool. It helps you to sort the real differences in opinion and conflicts that you experience with others from the ones that are based on your assumptions and expectations. Clear communication may also help to change a conflict that feels irremediable ("You always avoid me when I am in pain. I think you are insensitive...") to a problem that can be negotiated ("I want to help you, but I don't know how. When you are in pain, you stop talking and I feel powerless to help...").

Community Support

Crohn's and Colitis Foundations

There are several organizations in North America that, in addition to raising money for research, also provide education and support to patients and families. Two such organizations are the Crohn's and Colitis Foundation of Canada (CCFC) and the Crohn's and Colitis Foundation of America (CCFA). Although the national offices of these organizations may not provide individuals with the type of small group support and personal contact that they are looking for, the local chapters are often a good way to network with other patients and families dealing with IBD.

Internet Resources

The availability of other community support varies from location to location, but many patients and families turn to the Internet, where there are numerous means of communication with other individuals who are in situations similar to your own. However, you should be careful about the quality of the information and support that you might find in places like Internet chat rooms. Typically, these are not monitored by someone with the necessary expertise who can put the information and opinions provided into proper perspective or context. If you hear or read something unusual, something disturbing, or something that just doesn't seem right, you should discuss it with your doctor.

Opportunities for Kindness

Telling others about your disease can be a liberating, rather than an embarrassing, experience. Many people are sympathetic to your condition and respond to your confidence in them with acts of extraordinary kindness, as Robert Mason Lee, a celebrated author with Crohn's disease, observes:

"People are always telling me that because I have Crohn's disease I shouldn't be doing the fun things they are doing — like having a beer, for example, or eating something other than brown rice. It is hugely annoying, because almost without exception these people do not know what they are talking about, recommending foods I know would leave me in hospital or warning me away from foods that I enjoy. I do my best to forgive these people for their helpful instinct, because I understand the desire to heal...

"What I have found, instead, is that just about everyone is good at offering comfort. I have had the hands of compassion laid upon me by doctors, nurses, ambulance attendants, the women in my life, friends, the wives of friends, complete strangers in bus terminals. When it comes to offering solace, people have a natural ability which transcends social place or relationships. We just give, naturally, of ourselves to those in need.

"One small consolation of having such a painful illness is the many opportunities it allows others to show kindness; the one great reassurance is how seldom I have been disappointed."

Great Comfort

One of the things that you will probably realize soon after you find out that you have Crohn's disease or ulcerative colitis is that you are not alone. Many thousands of people have gone through experiences similar to your own. By linking up with some of these people, you may find a valuable source of information, as well as psychological and emotional support. Knowing that you not alone can be a great comfort.

In addition, remember that, although IBD is considered a single group of diseases, its presentation and response to treatment can be completely different from one person to the next. As a result, what one person experienced or a treatment that helped someone may not necessarily apply to you. These Internet sites do provide an opportunity for you to discuss your thoughts, feelings, and hopes with others, particularly if you find it difficult to do so face to face. The responses that you get may not always make you feel better, but, in many cases, people are able to find some comfort in describing their situation and knowing that there are others in similar situations.

Coping with the Medical System

Navigating through the medical system successfully can be a stressful challenge in itself. Having a chronic disease means that over time you will likely need to make use of a variety of medical resources, including hospitals, clinics, and laboratories.

Managing Medical Meetings and Appointments

Many people find medical visits to be stressful, especially when things are changing — when there are new symptoms or a new diagnosis, or a new treatment is being considered. Anxiety and stress make it harder to pay attention and take in all of the information that is being discussed. The stress of the situation also makes it harder to retain the composure that you need to ask your questions and make sure that they are answered.

Try to anticipate what you want to get out of a meeting with your doctor or specialist and prepare yourself accordingly.

• Make sure there is enough time. Make an appointment to address your concerns instead of trying to find a moment at the end of another conversation.

• Make a list of your questions. Keep it short enough that it can realistically be covered in the available time.

• Bring a friend or relative to help you remember what you have discussed.

• Make notes.

You are also likely to come in contact with a wide range of professionals in these settings — nurses, dietitians, enterostomal therapy nurses, family doctors, gastroenterologists, surgeons, emergency department staff, pharmacists, and many others are often helpful along the way. Some will be seasoned experts and some will be students full of enthusiasm and recent knowledge.

Communication and Coping Strategies

Treating pain appropriately is a common challenge for many people with IBD and may easily become a source of conflict and miscommunication with health-care professionals. Most medical care starts with a conversation in which patients try to explain their symptoms, while the doctor tries to listen, understand, and explain the available options. Then patient and doctor try to come to an agreement about how to proceed. Such a conversation amounts to a negotiation — and negotiations are difficult in a context of pain and stress.

Fortunately, when both parties negotiate in good faith, which is almost always the case, it is not hard to build an alliance and face the problem as a team.

Strategies for coping are also needed when you're undergoing drug and surgical treatments. Use your strengths to face these challenges. Others around you — friends, acquaintances, family members, or health-care professionals — will often be helpful if you are able to tell them what is wrong and how they can best help you.

Treatment Challenges

At times, getting the most comfortable and effective treatment for your IBD will challenge your ability to be an effective advocate for your own rights and interests, to work collaboratively with others (including times when there is disagreement), and to make the best use of the resources and supports that are available to you.

A Visit to the ER

To illustrate the complex forces that are at work between a patient and a doctor, imagine what looks on the surface to be a fairly straightforward case: Jane, who has Crohn's disease, goes to the emergency department because of intense abdominal pain. She wants to know what is going on and she needs relief. She is seen by Dr. Smith. This looks like a relatively uncomplicated medical situation, surely one that occurs quite often, but other factors make it a frustrating and difficult experience. Consider the following possibilities:

- Abdominal pain has been a chronic part of Jane's experience for years now. Although chronic pain hurts just a much as acute (sudden) pain, it doesn't look the same. People with chronic pain are not as likely to be pale and sweating, pacing or writhing, rocking in their seats, or making the noises that people with acute pain tend to make. The consequence is that Jane may not look like her pain is as severe as it feels.

- Jane has no way of knowing how the intensity of her pain compares to what other people experience. It is the nature of "invisible" symptoms that we have no objective yardstick to measure them. Many people are unsure of when to ask for help and when to tough it out. Unfortunately, these choices are heavy with value judgments. No one wants to be considered a wimp or a bother. But neither should anyone accept needless suffering. Jane may not be clear in her own mind that she deserves pain relief.

- Dr. Smith is well aware that there are a number of painful intestinal conditions that should not be treated with strong narcotic (opioid) pain medications, either because the drug masks the pain while the condition is getting worse (as can happen with undiagnosed appendicitis, for example, making it difficult for the health-care professionals to monitor the situation), or because the side effects of the drug can make the problem worse (as when pain medications prevent the bowel from functioning normally and aggravate an obstructed bowel).

- Dr. Smith is also aware that irritable bowel symptoms sometimes occur in the course of Crohn's disease, and so the flare of pain may or may not indicate that something has changed in Jane's gut (such as an increase in inflammation or an obstruction to the passage of the contents of the gut). Pain of that sort is called functional pain. He chooses his words carefully, because sometimes when he talks about the possibility of functional pain, his patients assume that he is telling them that the pain is "in the head."

- Dr. Smith has never met Jane before and has no way to judge her usual pain tolerance or how trustworthy she is in reporting her degree of pain. Trust is an important issue because the strongest pain medications are opioids, which can be abused and cause addiction. Jane has used opioids only once before, when she was recovering from surgery. She used them as prescribed and had no difficulty stopping them after a few days when they were no longer required. Dr. Smith doesn't know this.

- Jane has never met Dr. Smith before and does not know that he is quite familiar with Crohn's disease and the treatment that she needs. She was seen by a doctor at another emergency department previously, who was dismissive and didn't seem to appreciate her condition. Her expectations of this visit are shaped by that experience to some degree, and she is aware that she is more guarded and irritable than usual when answering Dr. Smith's first few questions. It feels like she is off to a poor start, which increases her tension.

- Dr. Smith is trying to balance a number of concerns. In addition to trying to provide the best care to Jane (and the other patients in the emergency department under his care), he has a professional and legal obligation to prescribe opioid medications responsibly. Unfortunately, it is a common experience in the emergency department for persons with addictions to exaggerate complaints in order to obtain opioids. Dr. Smith's expectations of this encounter are also shaped by previous experiences.

Neither Jane nor Dr. Smith is actually thinking about **all** of the considerations in this list. But they may all be at play.

How do Jane and Dr. Smith navigate through these tricky waters? Fortunately, if this encounter goes the way of most visits to the emergency department, they will be able to communicate effectively and Jane will get the help she needs quickly. Jane will be honest and open in discussing her concerns, her current situation, and her past experiences. Dr. Smith will listen carefully and be forthright about his reasons for choosing the investigations and treatments that he believes are indicated. As with most negotiations, mutual trust and respect are the bedrock of emergency room communication, and for both parties, the best way to receive them is to give them.

It may help Jane to bring a trusted support person with her to the emergency room, who can quietly support her efforts and act on her behalf if her pain interferes with her ability to speak or care for herself. A supportive person can also act as a "backup memory" when medical information is provided, because patients in distress often find it hard to remember new information. Also, just having a friendly third party in the room often helps to prevent Jane or Dr. Smith from falling into a trap of false expectations or assumptions that complicate their exchange.

CHAPTER 7

Drug Therapy for Managing IBD

CASE STUDY **Jonathan**

Jonathan, the police officer with suspected Crohn's disease, underwent a number of blood and stool tests, CT enteroclysis, and a colonoscopy. These investigations confirmed the presence of Crohn's disease involving the last part of the small intestine (ileum) and a small section of the large intestine (sigmoid colon). His doctor recommended drug therapy.

Jonathan was initially placed on budesonide and a combination of antibiotics (metronidazole and ciprofloxacin), but quickly developed a metallic taste in his mouth and persistent nausea. His gastroenterologist told him that this was probably occurring because of the metronidazole, and he advised him to cut the dose in half.

With this, Jonathan was able to continue the prescribed treatment, but though his symptoms improved somewhat, he was still experiencing episodes of mild pain and diarrhea at least 2 days out of every week and had not regained the weight he had lost.

Although the symptoms were not very bad and weren't really interfering with his work or his leisure time activities, even biking, he wondered whether he might do better with an alternative type of therapy.

He raised this question with his doctor, and they went through the available treatment options, ranging from steroids through immunosuppressive drugs to the newer biologic drugs. Jonathan had many questions about the likelihood of those medications providing him with additional benefit and their ability to change his long-term prognosis. He had already had the bad experience of a side effect from his relatively brief exposure to medication and was also concerned about the side effects and long-term safety of medications. Since he was feeling reasonably well at the time, he decided, after a full discussion of the available options, not to embark on any new treatment.

Medication Considerations

Making the decision to take drug treatment for IBD, as well as choosing what drug to take at what dose and for how long, can be very complicated. There is no standard treatment for IBD that is effective in all situations for all patients. Every patient and every situation is somewhat different. Decisions about medical therapy need to be tailored for each person to meet the nature of the disease, while taking into consideration personal circumstances. This typically involves consideration of the chance of improvement with therapy and the possible side effects or risks of therapy. For some people in countries, states, or provinces where medication is not paid for through private or public health insurance plans, the cost of the medication may also be a consideration in making treatment decisions.

Standard Treatments

The lack of a standard treatment for IBD is also due to the fact that IBD sufferers vary widely with respect to the form of IBD they have, the location within the gastrointestinal tract affected, the severity and aggressiveness of the disease, and the complications of the disease. Patients also vary widely with respect to the side effects they are willing to risk or able to tolerate. They may respond differently to the means of administering the drug — pills, liquid suspensions, injections under the skin, infusions into a vein, suppositories, or enemas. As a result, what might be the best treatment for one patient might not be the best treatment for another patient with the same disease severity, location, and complications. For some patients, surgery may be required; for others, symptoms can be treated with medications and surgery can be avoided.

Individualized Medication

The aggressiveness of the disease differs from patient to patient. Other differences depend on whether patients develop a complication of their disease, whether the disease location extends or becomes more widespread, and whether the inflammation becomes resistant to medical treatment.

Some patients with Crohn's disease have mild symptoms that respond extremely well to medical therapy and never progress to develop strictures, fistulas, or abscesses, whereas others seem to experience one or more of these complications within a matter of months or a few years. Because these complications often require surgery, it would seem to be even more important to effectively treat Crohn's disease in these individuals before the disease progresses to that point.

Similarly, some patients with ulcerative colitis first present with inflammation that is limited to the rectum and sigmoid colon only, with the remainder of the large intestine being unaffected. In the majority of these patients, the disease remains localized to that last part of the large intestine, but a minority do have progression to involve all or most of the large intestine, a potentially more serious situation. When a patient is first diagnosed with IBD, it would be extremely helpful to know what the likely course of disease will

Adapted Drugs

The development of new drug therapies for IBD has, until recently, been quite slow and, in most instances, the medications that have been used in IBD have not been specifically developed for the treatment of IBD. Instead, they have been adapted from use in other disorders.

be. This will, in turn, help physicians make recommendations regarding the best therapy for a given patient and will help the patient and her family make the best decisions for her situation.

Step-Up or Top-Down Therapy

Clearly, if a given patient has a very good prognosis, with only a small chance of developing complications of disease or requiring surgery, it would be best to treat her first with medications that have a lower likelihood of side effects but may be somewhat less potent or consistent in terms of treating inflammation. If these medications are not effective in controlling inflammation and the associated symptoms of IBD, then she could be considered for the more potent therapies that may be associated with a higher chance of side effects.

- **Step-Up Therapy:** This is a stepwise approach to treatment based upon response to the various available medications. It is still used in ulcerative colitis and has been the usual standard in patients with Crohn's disease.

   However, because of the potentially irreversible nature of the complications that can occur in Crohn's disease and the frequent need for surgery once they occur, there has been a move toward using the more potent and more consistently effective therapies earlier on in the course of the disease, before complications have occurred.

- **Top-Down Therapy:** Provided that treatments are effective and safe, readily available and not excessively expensive, this approach would seem to be the best for many patients with Crohn's disease.

Benefits vs. Risks Assessment

Any given person with IBD may be likely to respond positively to a given medication, but may not be willing to take the possible risk of certain rare serious side effects. Another person might be willing to accept a relatively high risk of side effects for the sake of receiving the most effective treatment. The final decision about medical treatment of IBD requires, under ideal conditions, a full discussion among the doctor, the patient, and, where necessary, the family.

In addition to non-steroidal anti-inflammatory drugs, there are other medications that are thought to have the potential to cause exacerbations or flares of IBD. Many of these medications are available only by prescription from a doctor. Every time you are given a new prescription, ask your doctor what the effect of the new medication might be on your IBD and if it has

---

Drug Guidelines

A number of different medical groups and societies have developed guidelines for the treatment of IBD. However, these guidelines are only general recommendations based upon the weight of evidence from clinical studies and from extensive personal experiences. They cannot reflect all of the subtleties and nuances of treatment in the individual patient and cannot be considered the standard treatment.

any interaction with the other medications you might already be taking for your IBD. Your doctor may not have an answer right away but will consult a reference source or ask a colleague with more experience. With the hundreds and hundreds of available medications, it is very difficult for any one individual to know about all of the possible interactions or effects of all of the medications.

Q What are side effects?

A Doctor and patient should assess the risks of drug therapy, not only the common and usually less serious side effects, but also the more rare and more serious potential side effects. Side effects can generally be divided into two categories – those that occur more often the higher the dose of the drug taken and those that are unpredictable and can occur at any dose of the drug. The first category of side effect may not occur in the majority of patients treated with the medication in the usual dose range, but tends to be more common the higher the dose used. These side effects can sometimes be dealt with by reducing the dose of the drug. The second category of side effects does not seem to occur more frequently at higher drug doses. These side effects appear to be similar to an allergic reaction and usually mean that the drug cannot be used any more because the reaction may occur even at low doses.

Similar to the way that physicians are trying to develop risk profiles for IBD complications that can be used in individual patients, there has also been work done in developing risk profiles for an individual's likelihood of experiencing a given side effect to a given drug therapy. A small number of these predictive tests currently exist. For example, a blood test can predict the chance that a given patient will develop a serious but rare blood complication of treatment with azathioprine (Imuran) or 6-mercaptopurine (Purinethol). If this blood test shows a low level of an enzyme involved in the metabolism of these drugs, then a patient is at increased risk of this blood complication and, as a result, can develop serious and life-threatening infections. If this blood test is performed before starting treatment and is found to be abnormally low, these drugs will usually not be considered as viable options or, if they are used, they will be given at very low doses.

However, in most instances there are no blood tests that will predict a high risk of side effects for most drugs used to treat IBD. As a result, doctors have to use other factors, such as a patient's age, to predict risk of side effects. It is clear that the risk of serious infection is higher in older patients treated with drugs that suppress the body's immune system as compared to younger individuals. This is why doctors are generally more reluctant to use immune suppressant medications in elderly IBD patients. The higher risk of this particular serious side effect may begin to outweigh the possible benefit of treatment.

Personalized Medicine

The type of treatment approach based upon individual patient prognosis or risk is often called "personalized" health care or "personalized" medicine. This is being touted as the best way to give the right therapy to the right patient at the right time so as to maximize the likelihood of beneficial short- and long-term effects while, at the same time, minimizing the risk of side effects or bad outcomes of treatment. On a societal level, this approach also ensures that the maximum benefit is achieved for the money spent on medical therapy for IBD by directing the most expensive treatments to the right patients based on their risk or prognosis.

Doctor-Patient Consultation

Some patients will ask the doctor, "What do you think is best?" and then trust the doctor to make the final recommendation on their behalf, based upon the doctor's knowledge and experience in treating IBD and any insight the doctor may have into the patient's individual circumstances and psychological makeup. Others may not be so compliant, finding that even an extensive discussion with the doctor about the treatment options is not sufficient. They will look for other sources of information, such as the Internet or other IBD patients, in order to try to make decisions for themselves. The reliability of these approaches to information gathering should be discussed with a health-care professional.

Drug Information Sources

Many physicians, clinics, and hospitals have preprinted sheets that outline the nature of the various medications used to treat IBD, including when they are to be used and what can be expected from their use, with information on how to recognize the possible side effects. Some pharmacies provide similar drug information sheets for patients at the time of drug dispensing. There are also some websites that offer similar drug information, but the quality of that information varies from site to site. If in doubt about the quality of the site and its information, check with your doctor.

Some medications also require specific monitoring with periodic blood tests, for example. The patient may need this information to make a treatment decision.

Whenever the treatment of IBD is discussed, the fact that it is a chronic and lifelong disorder must be considered. Although some medications may be very effective at controlling inflammation and symptoms for a short period of time — days or weeks — what is really needed are medications that can safely and effectively ensure that, once a disease flare is under control, the IBD sufferer will be less likely to experience a recurrence of disease flares.

Questions to Discuss with Your Doctor about Drug Therapy

- Is drug treatment of my IBD necessary?
- Is the treatment intended to bring a flare under control or is it intended to maintain a remission?
- What benefits can I expect from this treatment? What symptoms will improve and what symptoms are not likely to improve?
- How quickly can I expect to see an improvement?
- What are some of the common side effects?
- What are the serious side effects that can occur with this therapy?
- Are there any other options for drug therapy in my situation?
- What is the cost of treatment?
- How long will I have to be on therapy?
- Is surgery a viable option in my situation?

Drug Therapy Options

Recommendations for treatment are divided into broad categories. These categories are determined by two considerations: whether Crohn's disease or ulcerative colitis is being treated; and, within each disease, whether the aim is to bring a flare or symptoms of active disease under control or to keep a patient well once a remission has been obtained through whatever means necessary. In some instances, recommendations may be further subdivided according to the location of the disease within the gastrointestinal tract and the severity of a flare. Certain complications of the diseases, such as abscesses in Crohn's disease, may also be considered as belonging in another category of disease treatment. These categories may be important because, in the case of several medications, they appear to be effective only in very specific situations and not in other situations.

Each drug or category of drugs may be used for different indications within IBD. For example, antibiotics are typically

No One Drug

Currently, there does not appear to be any one medication that is effective for all forms of inflammatory bowel disease and for all of its complications.

not used in ulcerative colitis because they don't appear to be very effective, but in patients with Crohn's disease, antibiotics do appear to be effective and are often used to reduce pain, improve drainage, and reduce the risk of widespread infection when a complication, such as an abscess or fistula, has developed.

Non-steroidal Anti-inflammatory Drugs

In general, the class of medication that you should be most concerned about using is the non-steroidal anti-inflammatory drugs used for pain relief, because they may result in disease flares in some people with IBD. These include drugs with the generic names diclofenac, sulindac, naproxen, and ibuprofen, to name a few. Although most are available only by prescription, ibuprofen is available over the counter in Canada and the United States under many different brand names. Be sure to read labels on every over-the-counter medication you purchase, and if you're not certain about its impact on your condition, consult your pharmacist or doctor.

Pain Relief

Non-steroidal anti-inflammatory drugs are commonly used to relieve pain and as an anti-inflammatory for a variety of forms of arthritis. Although not every IBD sufferer will run into problems when taking non-steroidal anti-inflammatory drugs, a proportion find that they produce increased abdominal pain, diarrhea, and rectal bleeding. These drugs can be used in IBD patients if absolutely needed for the treatment of other forms of inflammation or sources of pain, but be certain that the indication for use is clear and that the treatment goals are equally clear so that therapy does not go on for any longer than necessary. Also consider other available alternatives that might be safer in IBD while achieving similar beneficial effects.

For relatively minor aches and pains, such as headaches, acetaminophen (Tylenol) is often effective and perfectly safe to take if you have IBD. If pain is more severe and an anti-inflammatory effect is not needed, then acetaminophen with codeine (for example Tylenol #2 or Tylenol #3) will provide pain relief without risk.

Narcotics

Chronic use of codeine and other narcotic medications, such as oxycodone (a component of Percocet) or meperidine (Demerol), can lead to addiction. They should only be used for episodes of acute pain (for example, after surgery) with a definite end point for completing therapy.

Pain Clinics

When someone with IBD has chronic pain that is not manageable through treatment of the underlying IBD or through simple non-specific measures, such as acetaminophen, then referral to a chronic pain clinic is indicated. These clinics usually have a team made up of anesthetists (pain specialists), physiotherapists, occupational therapists, psychiatrists or psychologists, social workers, and pharmacists with the goal of controlling pain in individuals with chronic pain syndromes. In some cases, they may also employ alternative practitioners, such as acupuncturists.

Commonly Used IBD Medications

Mesalamine (5-aminosalicylic acid) containing preparations
- Sulfasalazine (Salazopyrin, Azulfidine)
- Delayed-release mesalamine (Asacol, Pentasa, Salofalk, Mezavant, Lialda)
- Balsalazide (Colazide)
- Olsalazine (Dipentum)

Glucocorticoids (Steroids)
- Prednisone
- Budesonide (Entocort)
- Prednisolone
- Hydrocortisone
- Betamethasone (Betnesol)
- Methylprednisolone (Solu-Medrol)

Antibiotics
- Metronidazole (Flagyl)
- Ciprofloxacin (Cipro)

Immunosuppressants
- Azathioprine (Imuran)
- 6-mercaptopurine (Purinethol)
- Methotrexate
- Cyclosporine

Biologic Therapies
- Infliximab (Remicade)
- Adalimumab (Humira)
- Certolizumab pegol (Cimzia)

Mesalamine (5-Aminosalicylic Acid) Containing Drugs

Mesalamine (also known as 5-aminosalicylic acid or 5-ASA) has a chemical structure very similar to aspirin, but its medicinal properties are somewhat different. Unlike aspirin, 5-ASA is not a pain reliever, but it does appear to have many anti-inflammatory actions similar to aspirin, although its anti-inflammatory actions appear to be fairly specific to the intestinal tract. These anti-inflammatory activities in the intestinal tract are hoped for when medications containing 5-ASA are prescribed.

Taken as a pill or a powder, 5-ASA is very quickly absorbed from the upper part of the small intestine and it then enters into the bloodstream. However, for this drug to be effective, it has to be within the intestine and not in the bloodstream. Therefore, drugs containing 5-ASA that have been produced for IBD all have some way of keeping the 5-ASA within the intestine and preventing it from being absorbed before it gets down to the parts of the intestine most commonly affected by IBD.

Sulfasalazine

Sulfasalazine is composed of two parts — a sulfa antibiotic and 5-ASA — that are connected by a chemical bond. This bond is split by an enzyme produced by the bacteria present in the large intestine and the last part of the small intestine. This releases the sulfa antibiotic and the 5-ASA into the bowel, where they can act on the inflammation in the inner lining of the intestine. The beneficial action of sulfasalazine in IBD is primarily due to the 5-ASA part of the drug, although the whole intact drug, containing both salfa and 5-ASA, may also have some beneficial effect.

When a flare of ulcerative colitis or Crohn's disease is severe, sulfasalazine and other 5-ASA-containing drugs are usually not effective. Trying to use them may end up having negative effects because of a possible delay in starting stronger or more effective medications. In those situations, the inflammation has probably progressed beyond a point where sulfasalazine can be effective.

Side Effects

In a small but significant proportion of patients, sulfasalazine was found to have a number of troubling side effects, most commonly stomach upset, often with nausea and vomiting, especially when higher doses were used. Unfortunately, higher

Accidental Discovery

Sulfasalazine was one of the first drugs found to be effective in the treatment of Crohn's disease and ulcerative colitis. It was originally used to treat a form of arthritis, but was found by accident to be effective in people who had both arthritis and ulcerative colitis.

Sulfasalazine Benefits

- Sulfasalazine medication is effective in treating the symptoms of ulcerative colitis as long as the inflammation in the colon isn't too severe. It also helps to keep the disease in remission once a flare has come under control.
- Sulfasalazine is probably effective in milder flares of Crohn's disease, but mainly when the large intestine is affected. However, it seems to be less effective when Crohn's disease affects the small intestine. Sulfasalazine also doesn't appear to prevent flares in Crohn's disease the way it does in ulcerative colitis.

doses appear to be more effective than lower doses that have fewer problems with stomach upset.

There are other side effects that can occur — skin rashes, fever, decreased blood cell counts, and infertility in males. Most of these occur only rarely and are not related to the dose of the medication, but they can be very severe. They appear to be due to the sulfa part of the drug. Knowing about this difference in the impact of the two parts of the sulfasalazine molecule has allowed researchers to develop newer 5-ASA-containing medications that do not have the sulfa associated with many of the side effects of sulfasalazine.

Controlled-Release Mesalamine (5-ASA) Preparations

To solve the problem of the side effects associated with the sulfa part of sulfasalazine and to prevent the 5-ASA part from being released and absorbed too far up in the small intestine, preparations have been formulated that keep the 5-ASA in the intestine and only release it when it gets to an area of the intestine where it can have its maximum action. This delay in the release of 5-ASA is achieved through several different means.

Some preparations of 5-ASA are coated in a waxy film that dissolves and releases the 5-ASA when the acid within the intestine becomes sufficiently neutralized. Examples of this type of preparation are Asacol, Salofalk, Mezavant and Lialda. In Pentasa, the 5-ASA is present in hundreds of tiny granules within a tablet form designed to allow the 5-ASA to escape slowly over time as the tablet passes down through the small and large intestine.

Pentasa is also available in some countries as granules that can be mixed with fluids or food, thereby making them easier to ingest. The 5-ASA-containing preparations are typically taken between 2 and 4 times per day, but there is evidence that, in certain circumstances, the entire daily dose can be taken at

5-ASA Benefits

- The 5-ASA-containing drugs can usually be used at higher, more effective doses than sulfasalazine, enabling many patients to reach the higher doses required to treat their disease.
- The controlled-release 5-ASA medications are useful in milder flares of inflammatory bowel disease, particularly ulcerative colitis, and are helpful in reducing the risk of recurrent flares in patients with ulcerative colitis.
- When the 5-ASA drugs were first developed, it was hoped that they would provide a safe and effective alternative to steroid medications in patients with Crohn's disease. Unfortunately, they have not been found to be as effective in Crohn's disease as had been hoped for. Despite the fact that there is some controversy about their effectiveness in Crohn's disease, many physicians still elect to use 5-ASA drugs early in the course of the disease because of their excellent safety record.
- In some patients with Crohn's disease, particularly those with involvement of the large intestine and those with mild disease, the 5-ASA-containing drugs will sometimes produce a noticeable benefit without risking the side effects that might occur with the stronger drugs, such as prednisone or immunosuppressives.
- The 5-ASA drugs may also reduce the risk of recurrence of Crohn's disease following surgical removal of the affected segments of the intestine. They are particularly appealing in that situation when using a drug for a period of several years, because the 5-ASA drugs have a well-proven, long-term safety record.

once without causing any loss of beneficial effect and with no increase in side effects. This once-daily dosing is also effective with Mezavant, Lialda and Asacol.

Side Effects

With the elimination of the sulfa part of the drug, the 5-ASA preparations result in fewer side effects, such as nausea, indigestion, and vomiting. Some of the other side effects occasionally experienced by patients taking sulfasalazine, such as the decreased blood count and infertility in males, also do not occur with the 5-ASA drugs. Patients receiving 5-ASA-containing preparations can still experience side effects, but they are usually mild.

Headaches

Patients occasionally find that they cannot take the higher doses required to treat IBD effectively because of headaches. At lower doses, patients usually find that headaches do not occur. Fortunately, most patients do not experience headaches, even at very high doses of 5-ASA. This is different from sulfasalazine, where many patients experience some type of side effect when a high dose is given.

Allergic Reactions

The allergic type of reactions that can occur unpredictably at any drug dose can occur as a result of 5-ASA use. These are extremely uncommon with 5-ASA, but can be very serious. Two examples of this type of side effect are pancreatitis (inflammation of the pancreas gland) and pericarditis (inflammation of the sac around the heart).

Convenience

Because 5-ASA is a relatively mild anti-inflammatory, high doses of the drug are required in order to see a beneficial effect. As a result, patients who are taking 5-ASA-containing compounds usually have to take multiple pills in multiple doses. This is less convenient than other medications, which can be taken once per day or even once per week or once every few weeks.

Some of the companies that produce the 5-ASA-containing compounds have addressed this issue by making tablets that contain a large dose of the drug so that a fewer number of pills need to be taken. In addition, there is some evidence that these drugs may be able to be taken as little as twice per day or possibly even just once per day without losing the beneficial effect.

Balsalazide

Balsalazide (Colazide) is another drug in the 5-ASA category, similar to sulfasalazine, in that it contains 5-ASA chemically bonded to another molecule. This prevents the drug from being absorbed in the small intestine. When it reaches the large intestine, the 5-ASA is split from the carrier molecule by

> ### Long-Term Safety
>
> The long-term safety of 5-ASA is excellent, with virtually no long-term side effects reported other than extremely rare damage to the kidney.

Balsalazide Benefits

- Balsalazide is effective in treating mild flares of ulcerative colitis and in preventing relapses once the disease is in remission. It hasn't been tested adequately in Crohn's disease.
- High doses of balsalazide are usually well tolerated because the carrier molecule produces no significant side effects.

enzymes produced by bacteria in he large intestine, thereby allowing the 5-ASA to have its anti-inflammatory effect on the inner intestinal lining.

Side Effects

The possible side effects are similar to those of the 5-ASA-containing compounds.

Olsalazine

Olsalazine (Dipentum) is composed of two 5-ASA molecules that are chemically bonded to each other. The two 5-ASA molecules cannot be absorbed effectively in the small intestine, but are split apart by the action of an enzyme produced by bacteria in the large intestine.

Olsalazine Benefits

- Olsalazine is effective in preventing relapses once the disease is in remission.

Side Effects

Olsalazine is somewhat different from the other 5-ASA-containing drugs because in about 15% of people who take this medication, the two 5-ASA molecules bound together can irritate the lining of the small intestine, resulting in increased diarrhea. Obviously, this side effect can be confused with worsening of the IBD. Olsalazine can also produce the other side effects that are rarely seen with 5-ASA-containing drugs, but not any more commonly than is seen with the other 5-ASA preparations.

Mesalamine Enemas and Suppositories

In patients who have ulcerative colitis with the inflammation limited to the rectum and lower part of the large intestine, a very effective approach to treating the disease is to apply mesalamine (5-ASA) directly onto the inflamed intestinal lining by putting 5-ASA into an enema or a suppository. These types of enemas and suppositories are commercially available in many countries under a variety of brand names, such as Salofalk, Pentasa, Rowasa, Canasa, and Asacol.

Enemas

Most people think that an enema is used to treat severe constipation. Liquid (typically water) is put into the rectum and

Enema Option

While not an appealing prospect, most people will accept a course of enema treatment, especially if they know that it is more likely to make them better and to make them better more quickly than other approaches.

Mesalamine Enema and Suppository Benefits

- Mesalamine enemas or suppositories are considered to be the first choice of treatment for ulcerative colitis where the inflammation is limited to the rectum or to the lower part of the colon. These enemas or suppositories are more effective in that situation than the 5-ASA preparations taken by mouth.

- Mesalamine enemas and suppositories are also extremely safe, with virtually no risk of serious side effects.

is expelled soon after with feces. However, medicated enemas containing 5-ASA are designed to be held in the rectum and the lower part of the large intestine so that the medication within the liquid has a chance to coat the intestinal lining and produce its beneficial effects.

Steps for Administering an Enema

The mesalamine enema comes in a plastic bottle containing between 2 and 4 ounces (60 and 125 mL) of the medicated liquid. The bottle usually has a smooth, tapered tip that can be inserted into the anus, usually with the help of some lubricant or by moistening with water.

- Lubricate or moisten the anus.

- Lie on the left side with your knees tucked up toward your chest.

- Insert the tip of the bottle into the anus and squeeze the bottle so that the liquid is injected into the rectum and lower part of the colon. Try not to squeeze the entire contents of the bottle into the rectum too quickly.

- Stay on your left side for at least 15 minutes after taking the enema and, if possible, do not get up again after that. It is best if the enema can be kept in overnight, but this is not always possible for someone with active ulcerative colitis.

- If you have very severe inflammation of the rectum, you may begin to feel cramping and a strong urge to move your bowels soon after taking the enema. It may be possible to overcome this urge and cramping by lying still, taking deep breaths, and trying to relax.

- In some cases, the pressure and urgency may persist, preventing you from falling asleep. Ultimately, you may have to get up and move your bowels.

- If you cannot retain the enema overnight, then keeping it in for at least 1 to 2 hours should still provide some benefit.

Even when patients are willing to take a course of enema treatment, they may not be able to keep the enema in the rectum for long enough to allow it to be effective. This inability to hold the enema usually occurs because the rectum is inflamed and, as a result, is very irritable and sensitive. When the rectum is irritable, there is typically a strong urge to empty the bowels as soon as there is something in the rectum causing it to be distended or stretched. This may be stool or it may be the liquid from the enema. The longer the enema is held, the farther up the colon it tends to spread and coat the surface. In general, most enemas do not reach much above the sigmoid colon and, as a result, are not fully effective for half or more of patients with ulcerative colitis.

Enemas are usually prescribed to be taken once per day, in the evening, as the last thing you do before going to sleep. This helps to ensure that the enema is held in the rectum and colon as long as possible. Many patients with IBD are able to administer an enema themselves, but some do require assistance because it requires flexibility to insert the tip of the enema bottle or tubing into the anus.

Suppositories

Some people who cannot tolerate or retain enemas are able to keep a 5-ASA-containing suppository in the rectum long enough for it to have an effect. The suppository usually dissolves very quickly and leaves only a thick pasty material containing the medication. Suppositories are large capsules or tablets with one end rounded and tapered, which allows the suppository to be inserted through the anus into the rectum, where the suppository dissolves, releasing the active medication.

Suppositories should be taken at bedtime, although some doctors advocate taking them twice daily, in the morning and at bedtime, to improve effectiveness. Despite this, most studies show that one nighttime dose every day is equally as effective.

Glucocorticoid (Steroid) Medications

When a doctor has an IBD patient with very active or severe disease, steroids have traditionally been the drugs prescribed. There are a number of steroids available on the market, and although they have slightly different chemical forms, they all have similar actions in IBD, with the exception of budesonide.

Suppository Delivery

Suppositories typically deliver the 5-ASA only to the rectum and not higher up. However, the dissolved 5-ASA suppository does not cause much irritation of the rectum, usually resulting in much less cramping and urgency than a 5-ASA enema. When only the rectum is diseased (ulcerative proctitis), a suppository is probably the best way to administer 5-ASA medications.

Steroids have been used for many decades in the treatment of inflammatory bowel disease. For most of this time, they have been the most consistently effective class of medications, having the advantage over many other classes of treatment because they generally work very quickly and can be used in a wide variety of forms of IBD.

The steroid medications used to treat IBD should not be confused with the steroids that are often talked about and still sometimes used for enhancing performance in athletes or body builders — the anabolic steroids. In fact, the steroids used to treat IBD have the opposite effect, if taken for long periods, of causing a loss of muscle bulk and strength.

Oral Steroid Benefits and Drawbacks

- Oral steroids, such as prednisone, typically begin working very quickly. In many instances, patients begin to feel better within several days of starting treatment, although complete disappearance of symptoms may take several weeks. This rapid action is a very attractive property of steroids, differentiating them from several other classes of medications, such as 5-ASA, that tend to take significantly longer to take effect.

- Although steroids are generally quite effective for the treatment of IBD, they have two main drawbacks — their lack of benefit when used to prevent recurrence of disease flares once the disease has been brought into remission; and their potential for producing short-term and long-term side effects. Some of these side effects may not reverse or go away once the dose is reduced or stopped.

Oral Steroids (Prednisone)

The most commonly prescribed oral steroid in North America is prednisone. It is inexpensive, typically costing only a few cents per day, and very effective, but has the risk of serious side effects, some of which can be very troubling and, in some cases, irreversible. Approximately half of patients who take steroids experience at least one side effect. For most of those patients, the side effects are not severe, but there is a significant minority who find the experience of being on steroids so negative that it makes them decide to never take steroids again, no matter how bad their IBD gets.

Dosage Regimen

When taken in oral form, steroids can usually be taken once per day, typically in the morning. They do not necessarily have

Cold Turkey

Prednisone must not be stopped suddenly, or "cold turkey," once it has been taken for more than 10 to 14 days. You may experience feelings of weakness, light-headedness, muscle and joint pain, abdominal pain, and diarrhea if you stop prednisone too quickly.

to be taken with meals, although this may reduce some of the potential for indigestion that some patients experience while taking higher doses of the drugs. Steroids are usually taken in courses of treatment lasting from 2 to 4 months.

Patients with an acute flare of IBD are usually started on a relatively high dose — 40 to 60 mg of prednisone per day — and the dose is gradually tapered over a period of 2 to 4 months. Different doctors may recommend different tapering schedules, and there is no evidence that one approach is better or worse than another.

However, prednisone and other steroids should not be stopped suddenly once they have been taken for a period of more than 10 to 14 days. Although this type of slow tapering of prednisone may reduce the chance that the IBD flares again as the dose is reduced, it is probably just as important in preventing the symptoms of steroid withdrawal.

Common and Reversible Side Effects

The most common side effects of prednisone affect a person's appearance, including increased appetite and weight gain, swelling of the feet and hands, rounding of the face (so-called moon face), acne, and easy bruising. For people who are very concerned about their appearance or who depend upon their appearance for their livelihood, these may be unacceptable side effects.

Fortunately, these common side effects tend to go away as a person reduces the dose of prednisone and is able to discontinue it. However, it typically takes much longer for the effects to go away as compared with how quickly they may begin as a person starts taking prednisone.

Weight Gain

The weight gain often seen with prednisone treatment may also seem like a positive effect for patients with IBD, who often have problems with weight loss or keeping weight on. However, the weight gain that occurs in patients with IBD is not a healthy type of weight gain. Most of the weight that is gained on steroids tends to be due to an increase in fatty tissue rather than an increase in muscle or lean body mass. This increase in body fat may take quite some time — usually many months — to come off once a person stops taking steroids.

Steroid Side Effects

Common and Reversible
- Rounding of the face (moon face)
- Acne
- Weight gain
- Fluid retention
- Increased appetite
- Insomnia and sleep disturbance
- Easy bruising and poor wound healing
- Mood swings
- Increased energy

Uncommon and Possibly Irreversible
- High blood pressure
- Diabetes
- Cataracts
- Osteoporosis
- Avascular necrosis of hip or other joint

Mood Swings

Another side effect that may be very troubling to patients is the mood swings and sleep disturbance that may come with high doses of prednisone (usually 40 mg per day or more). Some patients describe feeling "high" or "energized" while on prednisone, and many find it very difficult to fall asleep and stay asleep. Although this may seem like a positive effect for some people, in the long term it can lead to increasing fatigue, diminished work or school performance, and even psychiatric disturbances.

Depression

Steroids may also lead to depression, particularly in people who have a prior history of depression before going on the medication.

Uncommon and Possibly Irreversible Side Effects

Fortunately, most of the side effects described above tend to go away as the dose of steroid is decreased or after the steroid is stopped altogether. However, there are a number of side effects that tend to occur when steroids are used chronically, for many months or years, or that tend to be irreversible and do not go away even after steroids are stopped. Some of these are very rare and unpredictable, whereas the risk of others seems to increase the longer steroids are used.

These side effects include loss of bone strength or density (osteoporosis), clouding of the lens in the eyes (cataracts), increased blood pressure, increased blood sugar (diabetes), increased pressure inside the brain, thinning of the skin, impaired healing of wounds or cuts, and increased susceptibility to certain types of infections. Some of these complications, such as cataracts, are irreversible, whereas others, such as high blood pressure, high blood sugar, poor wound healing, and increased risk of infections, may diminish in severity or go away entirely when steroids are tapered and stopped. There is currently no way to predict the occurrence of these side effects, but they tend to occur more often the higher the dose and the longer the use.

Hypertension and Diabetes

Steroids are more likely to cause an increase in blood pressure or blood sugar in someone who is already predisposed or at risk of developing hypertension (high blood pressure) or diabetes (high blood sugar), respectively. Although steroids can be used in people with hypertension or diabetes, special care and close monitoring is required and, in many cases, alternative medications are tried before considering the use of steroids.

Sleep Problems

The sleep problems can be minimized by taking the dose of steroids in the morning, although when the problem is severe, this may not help very much and sleeping pills are often not effective. In many cases, the only solution is reducing the dose and stopping the steroids.

Calcium Supplements

For patients who have normal bone density when they start on steroids, there is no single accepted way to reduce the risk of bone loss due to steroids. At a minimum, you should ensure adequate intake of calcium and vitamin D and, if it is not adequate, take supplementation. Dairy products are usually the main source of calcium, but many IBD patients avoid them. In those individuals, supplementation is very important.

Osteoporosis

The loss of bone density (osteoporosis) is something that tends to occur relatively slowly, although more rapid bone loss can occur in the first few months of steroid treatment. The use of a special X-ray called dual energy X-ray absorptiometry (DEXA) is a safe and accurate way of measuring bone density over time.

In IBD patients who already have reduced bone density when they are started on steroids, the use of bisphosphonates (etidronate, alendronate, and risedronate) is frequently recommended. These drugs are most effective when taken along with calcium supplements, and can sometimes result in an increase in bone density. This usually requires a specific schedule of bisphosphonate and calcium dosing, with careful monitoring by a doctor.

These particular bisphosphonates are taken in pill form by mouth and can produce irritation of the gastrointestinal system and associated symptoms, such as abdominal pain and diarrhea. This can make it difficult for some IBD patients to take these medications. However, there are some bisphosphonates, such as pamidronate, zoledronate, and ibandronate, that can be administered intravenously on a relatively infrequent basis — anywhere from once every 3 months to once per year — and do not have the same effect on the gastrointestinal symptoms.

Avascular Necrosis

One particular complication of steroid treatment that is particularly feared is avascular necrosis. This is a very rare and unpredictable condition that can occur without warning even after a relatively short course of steroid treatment. Avascular necrosis involves a loss of the normal blood flow to the end of a bone, resulting in collapse of the end of the bone, which leads to pain and chronic arthritis. It most commonly affects the hips, but can occur in many other joints, including the knees and shoulders. The risk of this complication occurring in someone receiving prednisone is very small — much less than 1 chance in 100. What makes the situation even more complicated is the fact that it appears that avascular necrosis can, in rare instances, be a result of the underlying IBD rather than steroid treatment.

There is no known way of predicting who might develop avascular necrosis, but there has been some suggestion from experts that treatment with bisphosphonates may reduce the risk of avascular necrosis.

MRI is probably the best test to diagnose avascular necrosis. When detected early, before collapse of the bone has occurred, avascular necrosis of the hip can be treated by a

---

Reducing Risk

Any unusual joint pain, particularly in the hips, in someone receiving steroids for IBD should be taken seriously and be investigated. Early detection of avascular necrosis in the hip through the use of X-rays, bone scans, or MRI (magnetic resonance imaging) may reduce risk of collapse of the bone and arthritis.

---

surgical procedure called a core decompression. This procedure involves putting a hole in the outer lining of the bone to allow the increased pressure present in the center of the bone to be released and normal blood flow to resume.

Intravenous Steroids

Although most steroid treatment in IBD is given as prednisone in a pill taken by mouth, steroids can also be given as an infusion into the vein (intravenous) in patients who are very sick with IBD and who require hospital admission for close monitoring and possible treatment of complications.

Hospitalized patients whose IBD flare comes under control with intravenous steroids will typically be switched over to prednisone taken by mouth shortly before they are ready to be discharged from hospital. Usually, they are put on a relatively high dose of prednisone — somewhere in the range of 50 to 60 mg per day — and the dose is gradually reduced over a period of 2 to 4 months.

Rescue Therapy

Several medical "rescue therapies" for patients not responding to a 5- to 10-day course of intravenous steroid therapy have been advocated as effective ways of avoiding surgery. Among these rescue drugs are cyclosporine and infliximab. It may be possible to predict which patients will not respond to the standard intravenous steroid treatment and to treat them early with rescue therapy rather than waiting 5 to 10 days. This may result in better outcomes and may reduce some of the possible side effects of extended treatment with steroids. Some patients with severe IBD flares who do not respond to intravenous steroids do not want to consider the use of "rescue therapy" and may opt instead for surgery as the most effective way of dealing with the acute problem.

Budesonide

Unlike other steroids given by mouth, budesonide is very quickly broken down into a by-product that has no side effects once it is absorbed into the bloodstream. The form of budesonide (Entocort) used in IBD is encased in a special coating designed to release the drug in the last part of the small intestine (ileum) and the first part of the colon (ascending colon), the areas most often affected in Crohn's disease. Budesonide has been formulated in a controlled-release preparation or coating that releases most of the drug into the colon, where it is effective in ulcerative colitis. This application is undergoing clinical testing and is not yet approved for this indication. However, it is available in some countries as an enema for the treatment of ulcerative colitis affecting the rectum and lower part of the colon.

Side Effects

Side effects can occur, particularly with higher doses taken for prolonged periods. The typical dose is 9 mg per day given as one dose, usually in the morning. Like conventional steroids, budesonide does not seem to be highly effective at keeping patients in remission once the acute flare has been brought under control, although some patients who respond to the acute treatment seem to remain well when kept on a slightly lower dose of 6 mg per day. Keep in mind that budesonide is a steroid and monitoring for complications and side effects, such as loss of bone density, is still necessary.

> ## Fewer Side Effects
>
> Budesonide is an oral steroid that is much less likely to produce the typical steroid side effects.

Budesonide Benefits

- When released, budesonide has a local effect on the inner lining of the intestine and results in decreased inflammation and improved symptoms. Any portion of the drug absorbed into the bloodstream then gets inactivated and side effects are unlikely to occur.
- Budesonide is effective in treating mild flares of Crohn's disease involving those parts of the intestine with much less risk of side effects than "conventional" steroids, such as prednisone.

Steroid Enemas and Suppositories

There are a number of different commercially available medicated enemas and suppositories that contain steroids. The most commonly used steroid for enemas is hydrocortisone (Hycort, Cortenema). As with 5-ASA, steroids can be formulated into suppositories to treat ulcerative proctitis (ulcerative colitis affecting only the rectum). In some countries, steroid foam enemas (Cortifoam) are available. These can have an advantage over standard liquid enemas that is similar to the advantages of suppositories — they are easier to hold for some people who cannot hold the liquid enemas.

Side Effects

Some patients who respond to steroid enemas need to keep taking them to keep the disease under control. In those instances, with particular steroids, such as betamethasone (Betnesol), it is possible

Steroid Enema and Suppository Benefits

- Steroid enemas are generally indicated for the treatment of active ulcerative colitis of the rectum and lower part of the colon, but are sometimes used for the treatment of Crohn's disease involving the rectum. Although steroids enemas are effective in ulcerative colitis, they are typically used in instances where 5-ASA (mesalamine) enemas have been tried and have been found to not be effective.

- Steroid enemas have an advantage over oral or intravenous forms of steroids because patients taking steroid enemas do not commonly experience significant side effects, for at least two reasons. First, the amount of steroid medication in the enema is generally much less than the amount taken when the disease is treated with medication taken by mouth. This lower dose may be effective because the drug is put directly on the affected area of intestine rather than acting indirectly after being absorbed from the upper small intestine into the bloodstream. Second, the drug in the enema may not be well absorbed through the lining of the rectum or colon and, as a result, will not have any effect throughout the body. The amount of steroid in the various enemas and the amount that gets absorbed into the bloodstream do vary quite a bit from enema to enema.

- In addition to being used to treat ulcerative colitis of the rectum and lower part of the colon, suppositories and enemas can be used in combination with oral 5-ASA or steroids. They can sometimes be helpful in reducing the inflammation that is present in the rectum more quickly than oral medication. This may be greatly appreciated by patients because the symptoms they experience from inflammation of the rectum (urgency to move the bowels, loss of control, a feeling of incomplete emptying after a bowel movement, and pain in the rectum) are some of the most troubling they may experience.

Intestinal Inflammation

Scientific studies offer evidence that normal intestinal bacteria contribute to intestinal inflammation. This theory fits well with the experience of doctors and IBD sufferers, who have observed the beneficial effects of antibiotics in some IBD situations.

to start seeing more of the common steroid side effects, such as acne, water retention, and weight gain.

Antibiotics

Some antibiotics appear to benefit patients with Crohn's disease, especially the antibiotic metronidazole (Flagyl). The next most commonly used antibiotic in Crohn's disease is ciprofloxacin (Cipro).

When antibiotics are used to treat infections, it is important that the indication for antibiotic use be clear. Antibiotics are active only against bacteria and are not needed for viral infections, such as colds or flus. They should not be prescribed unless there is a strong suspicion or confirmation of a bacterial infection.

In particular, antibiotics appear to be useful in Crohn's disease when the large intestine is involved or when complications, such as abscesses or fistulas, have occurred.

Antibiotics are not usually used for long-term maintenance treatment, but some patients have recurrent symptoms when antibiotics are stopped and seem to fare better if they are kept on continuous long-term antibiotic therapy, sometimes in relatively low doses.

Antibiotic Benefits

- Although the effectiveness of antibiotics in IBD is not proven or accepted by all doctors, most do believe that antibiotics are effective in selected individuals with Crohn's disease, but probably not in ulcerative colitis.

Side Effects

There is a common misconception that antibiotics cause flares of IBD. While this may not be true, there are certain side effects that can occur when using antibiotics to treat IBD.

Metronidazole

Metronidazole (Flagyl) can produce an effect on the nerves in the hands and feet leading to a sensation of numbness and tingling. If severe, this can lead to muscle weakness. If patients taking Flagyl drink alcohol, they might feel very bad and experience a reaction that may include weakness, sweating, and flushing. Flagyl appears to be safe to use during pregnancy, particularly when used for only a short course of 7 days.

Most of the side effects are seen more frequently when higher doses are used; accordingly, there has been a tendency away from prescribing high doses of metronidazole. Ciprofloxacin has been used in combination with metronidazole by many doctors. When ciprofloxacin is added to metronidazole, the dose of metronidazole can often be reduced so that the side effects are less likely to occur.

Ciprofloxacin

Ciprofloxacin is usually well tolerated and has very few obvious side effects. The most common is an increase in the amount of diarrhea, which is usually temporary and tends to decrease as the ciprofloxacin produces improvement in the disease. There are some concerns about women taking ciprofloxacin during pregnancy because of possible effects on cartilage and joint

Metallic Taste

Because of possible side effects, metronidazole cannot be taken by everyone. However, it is not known if lower doses are as effective as higher doses that produce more prominent side effects. The most frequent side effects are nausea, vomiting, and an unusual taste in the mouth. The unusual taste has been described as "metallic."

development in the fetus. For similar reasons, ciprofloxacin has usually been avoided in children.

Clostridium difficile Colitis

In rare cases, a secondary infection, called *Clostridium difficile* colitis, can occur in the large intestine during or after a course of antibiotics. This can lead to large amounts of watery diarrhea and an exacerbation of underlying IBD. The antibiotics that are most commonly linked to *Clostridium difficile* infection are clindamycin and amoxicillin, although it has been described following virtually every available antibiotic.

Immunosuppressant Medications

Immunosuppressant medications cause some suppression of the body's immune response, which may be beneficial in IBD because the disease involves overactivity or overresponse of the body's immune system to something in the body or in the surrounding environment. The immunosuppressant medications used most commonly to treat IBD are azathioprine, 6-mercaptopurine, methotrexate, and cyclosporine.

In order to be useful, immunosuppressant medications must be used within a very narrow range of immune suppression so that patients do not become overly susceptible to infections. Even when used in appropriate doses, these drugs do increase the risk of certain types of infections, usually to a small extent, which varies from drug to drug.

Azathioprine and 6-Mercaptopurine

The value of azathioprine (Imuran) and 6-mercaptopurine (Purinethol) in treating IBD has been increasingly recognized since they were first used in the 1960s and 1970s. Although they are different drugs, they work in the same way and are considered to be interchangeable. Azathioprine and 6-mercaptopurine (6-MP) are given in pill form, taken once a day.

Long-Term Treatment

Azathioprine and 6-mercaptopurine are very slow-acting medications with respect to their beneficial effects. Once they are started, it usually takes 3 months on average for them to take full effect. As a result, they are not useful for treating acute flares of IBD, since most patients who are experiencing symptoms of active disease cannot wait for 3 months for their symptoms to improve.

When an IBD sufferer is started on azathioprine or 6-MP, it is usually with the understanding that it is a long-term treatment strategy — typically 3 or 4 years or more. Knowing whether or when to stop azathioprine or 6-MP in individuals who have responded well to them is extremely difficult. Most experts suggest that a minimum of 4 years is required before stopping therapy in someone who has done well. However, if there have been minor flares despite azathioprine or 6-MP therapy, it is likely that more severe flares will occur if the drug is stopped even after 4 years or more of therapy.

Azathioprine and 6-Mercaptopurine Benefits

- Azathioprine and 6-mercaptopurine are useful for keeping patients in remission and reducing the need, over time, for other medications, such as steroids.
- The effectiveness of these drugs in Crohn's disease is well accepted, but they are also being increasingly used in ulcerative colitis.
- They also appear to be safe in children, where they are increasingly used in order to avoid the need for repeated courses of steroids.
- There are reports of many women who have taken azathioprine or 6-MP during pregnancy without any bad effects on either the course of the pregnancy or on the baby. However, it is still not possible to completely prove that these drugs are safe in pregnancy, and any consideration of using them during pregnancy requires a careful and complete discussion between a woman and her doctor about the risks of continuing and the risks of stopping the medication.
- Azathioprine has also been found to be effective in Crohn's disease when used in combination with one of the newer biologic drugs, infliximab (Remicade). When used in people who have not had Crohn's disease very long and have not been previously treated with immune suppressants, the combination of azathioprine and infliximab is more effective than either drug given alone. Whether this benefit of combination therapy extends to the use of other biologic drugs, such as adalimumab (Humira), has not been specifically tested. In ulcerative colitis it appears that the combination of azathioprine and infliximab may offer an advantage over either therapy alone, but this is far from settled.

Side Effects

Although they require ongoing monitoring of blood tests, azathioprine and 6-MP are generally very well tolerated. A very small number of people experience nausea or gastrointestinal upset, but most patients experience no side effects that would make them aware that they are even taking medication. There are rare serious complications, however.

Allergies

Allergic reactions can occur, showing up as fever, skin rash, and worsening of IBD symptoms.

Abnormal Liver Blood Tests

Abnormal liver blood tests can also occur. Most often this does not occur with any symptoms and, as a result, requires monitoring of blood tests to detect. These abnormalities may be due to inherited differences among people in the way these drugs are metabolized and may improve with changes in drug dose. Liver blood test abnormalities may also be related to allergic reactions.

Pancreatitis

Azathioprine and 6-MP can result in pancreatitis (inflammation of the pancreas) in approximately 3% of patients receiving the medications. This is a potentially serious side effect that frequently requires hospitalization. In general, if pancreatitis does not occur in the first few weeks of treatment, it does not occur at all. If it does occur, it means that azathioprine or 6-MP cannot be used again for that individual.

Infection and Bleeding Complications

The dose of azathioprine or 6-MP initially prescribed for an individual patient is calculated based upon the patient's weight. However, because of the differences in drug metabolism from person to person, the dose may have to be modified based upon blood testing. When the dose of drug is too high for a given individual, the bone marrow's production of white blood cells (cells that help fight infection) and platelets (cells that are important in blood clotting) may decrease, leading to an increased risk of serious infection or bleeding complications.

If the levels of these cells get too low, the dose of the drug usually needs to be reduced or, in some cases, the drug must be stopped. Measuring the numbers of white blood cells and platelets in the blood is an easy and inexpensive way of monitoring the effect of azathioprine and 6-MP on the bone marrow. However, they are only indirect measurements of how much of the active by-product of the drugs reaches the bloodstream. More recently, other blood tests have been developed to directly measure the level of the active drug by-products in the bloodstream. This may allow more precise monitoring of drug dosing, but it has not yet been adopted into routine practice by most doctors.

Monitoring

Ongoing monitoring of blood tests is required as long as someone is taking azathioprine or 6-mercaptopurine. Initially, this may be as frequently as once per week, but for patients who have been on a stable dose without any abnormalities on blood testing, they can probably be checked once every 2 to 3 months. The ongoing monitoring is necessary because abnormalities can happen after many months or even years of being stable on the medication.

Thiopurine Methyltransferase Enzyme

There is another blood test that measures thiopurine methyl-transferase (TPMT), a key enzyme that determines how much of the active by-product is made for a given dose of the drug. This enzyme is abnormal or absent in a very small proportion of people (approximately 1 out of every 300 people). People who are lacking this enzyme produce very high levels of the active by-product and are at risk of developing severe reductions in white blood cells and platelets.

If patients are tested for this enzyme and found not to have it, they should probably not be treated with azathioprine or 6-MP or should be treated with very low doses. This blood test is still not used by many doctors because it is not widely available. What is often done instead is that the drug is started at approximately half of the dose that is calculated likely to be needed, and the white blood cell count and platelet count are closely followed for several weeks. If there is no sudden drop in the counts, the dose is then increased up to the target dose and the blood tests are continued to be followed closely.

Even if the white blood cell count remains normal for the first months after a person is started on azathioprine or 6-MP, a drop in the count can occur at any time during treatment. Although the risk is much lower than during the first few months, ongoing checking of blood tests is necessary as long as the person is taking the medication.

Cancer Risk

One of the most difficult issues for patients and doctors when considering the use of immunosuppressants, such as azathioprine and 6-MP, is the potential for future development of cancer. Any time there is suppression of the immune response, there is a theoretical increase in the risk of developing cancer. This has been extensively examined in patients who have been treated with azathioprine and 6-MP. Overall, it appears that the use of these drugs in IBD does not increase the risk of cancer, with the possible exception of lymphoma, a rare form of cancer of the lymph glands.

Not a Cure

Although these drugs may be effective at controlling disease symptoms over many months or even years, they are not cures for IBD. When treatment is stopped, the disease can recur and flare up with symptoms coming back, sometimes worse than prior to first starting immune suppression therapy. As a result, many doctors are reluctant to stop treatment in someone who is doing well, even when it has been more than 4 years. Certainly,

Minimal Risk

Although the use of azathioprine or 6-MP may increase the risk of lymphoma, the risk to any given individual taking these medications is extremely small. It has been calculated that azathioprine would need to be taken for more than 4,300 years for someone between the ages of 20 and 29 before observing one extra case of lymphoma. The risk of other cancers is not different in people taking azathioprine or 6-MP than in individuals not taking one of these drugs.

if there has been any sign of ongoing inflammation despite the fact that a person has had no significant symptoms, it is probably not wise to consider stopping therapy.

Methotrexate

Methotrexate was originally used to treat certain types of cancers. It interferes with the production of the genetic material, DNA, which, in turn, reduces the formation of new immune reactive cells, resulting in immunosuppression. Methotrexate may also have some anti-inflammatory action that may make it even more beneficial in IBD.

Now, methotrexate is used much more commonly in the treatment of chronic inflammatory disorders, such as rheumatoid arthritis or Crohn's disease, than in the treatment of cancer. To treat inflammatory disorders, methotrexate is usually taken once per week, either by mouth or by injection under the skin or into a muscle.

Methotrexate Benefits

- Methotrexate is used in many of the same situations as azathioprine and 6-MP.
- It is effective in treating active Crohn's disease that has not adequately responded to steroids, such as prednisone, and, once the disease has been brought under control, is helpful in keeping the disease in remission and avoiding repeated treatments with steroids.
- It is not clear whether methotrexate is effective in ulcerative colitis.
- In patients with rheumatoid arthritis, methotrexate is often given in combination with biologic drugs, such as infliximab (Remicade), where it has been consistently shown to increase the effectiveness of these drugs. This same strategy has not been shown to be effective in Crohn's disease, although the use of methotrexate does seem to lower the amount of antibodies that form against infliximab. These antibodies are potentially important because they can increase the possibility of side effects from infliximab and may reduce its effectiveness. However, this lower rate of antibodies against infliximab has not translated into better effectiveness with methotrexate. As a result, azathioprine or 6-mercaptopurine are generally the first choice for use in combination with infliximab in most situations.

Side Effects

Methotrexate is usually well tolerated, although some people experience nausea and sometimes vomiting. This typically occurs on the day of the week when the methotrexate is taken.

This side effect can usually be avoided or reduced by taking the drug in the evening before bed, by taking a supplement of the vitamin folic acid on the day that methotrexate is taken, or by taking an antinausea medication.

Liver Damage

Monitoring of liver blood tests is necessary while a patient takes the drug because methotrexate can result in liver damage and scarring. If the tests are abnormal, the drug has to be stopped or the dose reduced. The risk of liver damage may be increased by moderate to heavy alcohol consumption. The risk seems to increase the longer a patient takes the medication. Monitoring of the blood counts is also required, as it is for azathioprine or 6-MP, but the drug can usually be started at the indicated dose without significant risk.

Allergic Pneumonia

Another side effect that may be rarely experienced in patients receiving methotrexate is allergic pneumonia. If a patient taking methotrexate experiences coughing and shortness of breath, further investigation is usually necessary to look for possible pneumonia.

Cyclosporine

Cyclosporine is a very potent immunosuppressant medication often used in transplant patients to prevent rejection of the transplanted organ. It has been tested in both ulcerative colitis and Crohn's disease. While cyclosporine appears to have no role in the treatment of Crohn's disease, it does bring severe disease flares under control in ulcerative colitis.

Treatment Regimen

Cyclosporine is usually given at first as a continuous intravenous infusion. The intravenous treatment is kept going until the patient begins to improve significantly or until it is clear that the patient is not improving and surgery is needed to manage the flare.

When a patient improves significantly on intravenous cyclosporine, this drug is switched to a form that is taken by mouth (Neoral) instead of by intravenous. Once the patient is improving and is on oral medications, she is discharged from hospital and Neoral is continued for approximately 3 to 6 months. In most instances, azathioprine is started when the patient is discharged and it is continued after Neoral is stopped, in order to keep the disease in remission.

Cyclosporine Benefits

- Studies have consistently shown that cyclosporine is effective in bringing severe disease flares under reasonable control in ulcerative colitis.
- Cyclosporine is an option for patients who have tried most of the other medical treatments for their disease and found them either unsuccessful or unacceptable because of side effects.
- Cyclosporine is used almost exclusively in hospitalized patients with severe attacks of ulcerative colitis, usually when they have not responded to a course of treatment with intravenous steroids.
- Cyclosporine may "buy" patients some time to get the disease under better control before surgery, even if only temporarily, to get out of hospital, and to think more about the options available to them. In general, people feel better about their decisions, whether it is to go for surgery or to continue trying medical treatment, if they have some time to reflect and if the decisions are not made under duress.

Last Resort

Cyclosporine is not used early in the treatment of ulcerative colitis due to its potential to cause serious side effects. Even with the best medical treatments to maintain remission, approximately 50% of patients who require cyclosporine to bring a severe flare under control end up needing surgery within 1 year.

Side Effects

Cyclosporine should only be prescribed by doctors who are familiar with its use and know how to monitor patients receiving it and what side effects to look for. Serious infections and kidney damage are possible serious side effects. Other side effects from cyclosporine use are high blood pressure, tremor, seizure, and increased hair growth (not usually in places where you want hair to grow).

Serious Infections

As with other immunosuppressant medications, cyclosporine can increase susceptibility to infections. This appears to be more so with cyclosporine than with many of the other immunosuppressant medications.

There are cases of patients developing unusual or rare infections that would not otherwise be seen in someone whose immune system is not being suppressed. Some of these infections can even be fatal, particularly if not detected and treated early. They can occur without a reduction in the white blood cells that help to fight infection. As a result, monitoring the white blood cell count on blood testing cannot predict who will run into this type of complication.

Kidney Damage

When cyclosporine is given, it is usual practice to monitor the levels of the drug in the bloodstream. This is done on a daily basis when the treatment is first started, and although it can be done less frequently once a patient is switched to the capsule form, it must still be continued as long as a patient is receiving the medication. Monitoring the blood levels is important in reducing the risk of kidney damage from the cyclosporine, but it is not a guarantee.

Biologic Drugs

Infliximab (Remicade)

Infliximab is the first of a new class of drugs sometimes referred to as "biologics" or "designer drugs" developed in the lab and introduced in humans in a way different from traditional therapies. These drugs are designed either to block specific molecules or receptors on cells that are important in promoting intestinal inflammation or to activate other molecules or receptors that are key players in reducing intestinal inflammation. They have the potential to provide very targeted treatment. The hope is that by providing targeted treatment, the overall number of side effects will be reduced when compared to traditional therapies.

Infliximab is an antibody, produced using genetic technology, composed of part human protein and part mouse protein. It attaches to and inactivates a protein called tumor necrosis factor alpha (TNF-alpha). TNF-alpha is a critically important protein in the process of causing inflammation. Blocking its action results in improvement in intestinal inflammation and improved symptoms of IBD.

Treatment Regimen

Because the infliximab antibody is itself a protein, it cannot be taken by mouth because it would be broken down and made inactive by the digestive enzymes in the stomach and small intestine. Rather, it is given as intravenous infusions, usually over a period of 2 to 3 hours, in an infusion clinic or other out-patient facility.

The initial course of treatment prescribed may vary from physician to physician. Some prescribe one or possibly two infusions given 2 to 4 weeks apart and then assess the response to treatment before deciding on the usefulness of further treatments. Others give a "standard" three-dose "induction regimen" involving an initial infusion, a second one 2 weeks later, and a third one 4 weeks after the second. Following the third infusion, the response is assessed and further treatment decisions made.

Adamlimumab and Certolizumab

These relatively new biologic drugs act much like infliximab. Consult with your gastroenterologist to determine which biologic drug might be best for managing your IBD.

First Biologic Therapy

Infliximab is very effective in treating several forms of IBD. Infliximab is the first biologic therapy that has been approved for use in IBD: it was approved for use in Crohn's disease in 1998 in the United States and in 2001 in Canada and for use in ulcerative colitis in the United States in 2005.

Once an IBD sufferer has responded to an initial course of infliximab, repeated dosing with infliximab — usually every 6 to 8 weeks — will help maintain the initial improvement.

We know from clinical trials that infliximab continues to reduce the risk of relapse or flare for at least 1 year after treatment is first started. Although there is really no information from the clinical studies about what happens after 1 year, it has been the experience of many doctors treating patients with infliximab that flares tend to occur more often if the treatment is stopped even after 1 year.

The response to infliximab can be very impressive, and it may seem that the disease has been "cured," but once infliximab is stopped, the risk of recurrent symptoms goes up. There does not appear to be a clear "exit strategy" for the majority of patients when infliximab treatment is started. This may be difficult for both patients and doctors to accept, but the fact that Crohn's disease and ulcerative colitis are chronic disorders and that infliximab is a treatment and not a cure must be kept in mind. It only works as long as it is taken.

Antibodies

Some patients receiving infliximab will develop antibodies directed against it after receiving several doses. In some cases where antibodies form, there is a decrease in the length of time of the perceived beneficial effect.

Initially, the beneficial effect of an infusion may last for 8 weeks before symptoms start to recur, but when antibodies to infliximab develop, this may drop down to 6 weeks or even 4 weeks. In some instances, infliximab appears to stop working altogether. In those cases, using another TNF-alpha blocker that is entirely human protein — and presumably would not be blocked by antibodies against infliximab — may be effective at regaining a beneficial effect.

Currently, adalimumab (Humira) is the only completely human TNF-alpha antibody available in the United States and Canada.

Short-Term Safety

Since its release, infliximab has been used extensively throughout the world, not just in IBD but also in rheumatoid arthritis and a number of other disorders. The short-term safety record has been excellent. This is not to say that there aren't potential side effects, but these tend to be relatively rare events or relatively mild and easily manageable.

Infliximab Benefits

- In clinical trials, infliximab was first found to be effective in treating symptoms of active Crohn's disease: 60% to 80% of patients responded positively. Improvement appears to occur very quickly in many patients, often within days of a single dose, with patients sometimes experiencing an improvement in their overall sense of well-being, energy, and appetite within hours of a dose.

- Many of the patients who were first studied in the clinical trials were on other medications for their Crohn's disease — 5-ASA drugs, steroids, or immunosuppressants — and had not noticed a significant response to these treatments until they were given infliximab. These patients, sometimes described by physicians as "treatment resistant," pose the greatest challenge to doctors treating Crohn's disease. These are the patients who most frequently require hospitalization and surgery.

- Infliximab has also been found to be effective in the treatment of fistulas due to Crohn's disease. Previously, there was no proven effective treatment for this troubling complication, although antibiotics can often reduce some of the pain and drainage over the short term. Infliximab is the first treatment shown to cause fistulas to stop draining, and, with repeated dosing, infliximab can prevent drainage from recurring. Whether the fistulas treated with infliximab actually heal (that is, the channel actually closes up) or just stop draining, with the channel remaining present and open, is a matter of considerable controversy. However, from a patient's perspective, the distinction is not pressing since the important outcome is the elimination of pain and drainage from the fistula.

- When it was first found to be effective in Crohn's disease, there was considerable optimism that it would also be effective in ulcerative colitis. While the early studies of infliximab in ulcerative colitis were inconclusive, two recent large studies appear to show a beneficial effect in patients with active ulcerative colitis who have not responded to other ulcerative colitis treatments — once again, the "treatment resistant" patients. It appears that ongoing repeated dosing every 8 weeks helps maintain the initial improvement that is seen with infliximab in about 60% of patients.

Infusion Reaction

The most common side effect is an acute reaction that occurs in 5% to 10% of patients during the infusion process, most commonly experienced as flushing, warmth, and redness along with a feeling of chest tightness and shortness of breath. This does not appear to be an allergic reaction, but may be related to how quickly the medication is infused.

Although the reaction may be quite distressing, it is never serious or life-threatening. This reaction always goes away after stopping the infusion temporarily and administering an antihistamine or acetaminophen (Tylenol). Once the reaction has been settled, the infusion can be resumed at a slower rate. As the infusion progresses, the speed of the infusion can usually be increased again. These reactions can be prevented by antihistamine or steroid premedication taken just prior to the infliximab infusion.

Infections

Infliximab may affect the immune system in a way that makes a person more susceptible to certain infections, most notably tuberculosis. Soon after infliximab was approved for use in Crohn's disease and rheumatoid arthritis, a number of cases of tuberculosis were noted in patients receiving this treatment. Many of these cases occurred within 3 months of starting infliximab. Once this was recognized, patients embarking on infliximab treatment have commonly been tested for tuberculosis by means of a skin test and possibly a chest X-ray. If tuberculosis is detected, treatment of the tuberculosis is generally recommended prior to starting infliximab. This has resulted in a significant reduction in the rate of tuberculosis, back down to the rate that was observed before infliximab was introduced on the market.

Long-Term Safety

Although most physicians caring for IBD patients in any significant numbers feel comfortable with the short-term safety record and the potential benefits of infliximab and other commonly used TNF-alpha blockers, such as adalimumab (Humira), there are still some reservations about the possibility of long-term effects that will only become apparent after many years of use.

Infliximab was first used in clinical trials in the mid-1990s, and as a result there is some reasonable long-term follow-up on many patients to provide us with some early long-term safety information. At this time, there is no conclusive evidence that infliximab produces an increase in late effects, such as cancer. Nevertheless, in the United States, infliximab has been given a label that indicates an association with an increased risk of lymphoma, a relatively rare form of cancer of the lymph glands. Although there is no direct proof that infliximab carries this risk, there is evidence that other drugs designed to block the action of TNF-alpha may increase the risk of lymphoma in patients with rheumatoid arthritis. To some extent, this is akin to "guilt by association." The complete story will take several years to unfold, but there is currently no reason to avoid the use of infliximab due to a theoretical risk of lymphoma.

Due Caution

There may still be other unusual infections that can occur in patients receiving infiiximab and that cannot be screened for by means of skin tests or chest X-rays. Every patient receiving infliximab should report to a doctor any unusual symptoms, such as a cough or severe and persistent headache, especially if they are associated with a fever.

Adalimumab (Humira)

Currently, there is one completely human TNF-alpha blocker, adalimumab (Humira®), that is widely available and approved for the treatment of Crohn's disease. Adalimumab is an antibody against TNF-alpha that, unlike infliximab, which contains some mouse protein, is an entirely human antibody. When given to an individual, the adalimumab antibody is still seen by the immune system as being "foreign" and, as a result, can still cause formation of antibodies against the drug. However, the formation of antibodies against the drug appears to be less frequent with adalimumab than with infliximab. Like infliximab, adalimumab is effective in the short- and long-term treatment of Crohn's disease and in some patients with ulcerative colitis.

Because adalimumab is not given by an intravenous infusion, it does not carry the risk of an infusion reaction as does infliximab. However, there is sometimes some local pain and redness at the site of adalimumab injection. This occurs only in a small minority of patients and is usually mild and not long-lasting.

Convenience

Unlike infliximab, which is given by an intravenous infusion, adalimumab is given by an injection under the skin every 1 to 2 weeks. As a result, it offers some advantages in terms of convenience for patients who can be taught to do the injections themselves rather than having to go to a clinic or hospital where the infusion of infliximab is given.

Certolizumab pegol (Cimzia)

Certolizumab pegol is a biologic therapy that was developed to block the action of tumor necrosis factor alpha, similar to infliximab and adalimumab. It is different from these two drugs in that it is not a complete antibody but is only a fragment of an antibody that is attached to a large molecule called PEG in order to slow down its elimination from the body. It is given by subcutaneous injection, similar to adalimumab, initially three times over a 4 week period, and then once every 4 weeks. It has been shown to be effective in Crohn's disease treatment but has only been approved for use for this indication in the United States and Switzerland.

Other Biologic Therapies

There are many types of biologic therapies other than infliximab, adalimumab, and certolizumab pegol currently in various stages of development. Some of these will likely prove to be effective in IBD and sufficiently safe to allow them to be approved for use. Given the major step forward that occurred with the introduction of infliximab, there is great anticipation that future biologic therapies will provide similar advances in treating IBD effectively and safely, resulting in less need for hospitalization and surgery and improved quality of life for IBD sufferers.

Q I have been approached by my doctor to participate in a research study. What's involved in participating in a study? Should I do it? If I do participate, will I be a "guinea pig"? If I don't do it, will my doctor be upset with me?

A Clinical research in IBD is a critically important type of research that is aimed at finding and developing new and better treatments for IBD. It can also help to determine which treatment, among a variety of existing or available treatments, is the best treatment in a given situation. Clinical research is also needed by pharmaceutical companies in order to get a new drug approved for use for a given disease indication. If a cure for IBD is discovered in a laboratory where it has been developed and tested in mice, it will ultimately have to be tested in humans with IBD.

There are no wrong or right reasons for you to participate in clinical research. People participate in clinical research for a variety of reasons. Some want to have a chance to try new therapies that they normally wouldn't otherwise have access to because the therapies are not yet approved for use or because of prohibitive cost. Others want to advance research in the field so that others can benefit from the new knowledge that will be obtained from the study. Some people like the close follow-up and monitoring and quick and easy access to the health-care team that is typically provided as part of a clinical trial.

Clinical Research Study Designs

Blinded Trials

Quite often the study participants and the doctors are "blinded" to the study group assignment – that is, they do not know which group an individual has been assigned to. This blinding is maintained by using "dummy tablets" or placebos that are designed to look exactly like the drugs being tested. If you participate in this type of study and if the blinding process is working, you should not be able to know whether you are receiving the standard therapy or the experimental therapy.

There are a variety of different clinical study designs, but the most commonly used one is the randomized controlled trial. In this type of study, patients with a given condition (for example, Crohn's disease) are randomly assigned (such as by the flip of a coin) to receive either the "standard therapy" or the "experimental therapy." The patients are then closely watched for a period of time and the outcomes of interest are measured or monitored. An outcome may be, for example, elimination of all symptoms of Crohn's disease. By comparing the proportion of individuals receiving standard therapy and the proportion of individuals receiving experimental therapy who experience elimination of their symptoms, research scientists can make a conclusion about which one works better.

Risk

By definition, you are being experimented upon in this type of trial, but safeguards are put in place to protect your safety. Nevertheless, there is always some inherent risk in participating. This risk should be fully described to you in a patient information and informed consent document, which you will sign before the study begins. This document describes what the study is; who is carrying it out; why it is being carried out; what is involved in participating (for example, number and types of visits, procedures, and tests); what are the potential risks to you in participating; what are the potential benefits to you; what your rights are within the study; and what your rights are should you choose not to participate.

After reading the document, which can often be quite lengthy, you will have the opportunity to ask questions of the study coordinator or the study investigator. If you need to, you can take the document home so that you can look it over again and, if necessary, discuss the study with your family and friends or with another doctor. Before agreeing to participate in a study, you should be comfortable with the decision.

Obligation

You should not feel obliged to participate in the study, and a decision not to participate should not affect the health care that you receive from your doctor. Similarly, if you decide at any point during the course of a clinical study that you no longer wish to participate, your care will not be affected.

Questions to Ask

- What is the purpose of the study?
- Why do researchers believe the new treatment being tested may be effective?
- Has it been tested before?
- What kinds of tests and treatments are involved?
- How do the possible risks, side effects, and benefits in the study compare with my current treatment?
- What are the alternative treatments that are available to me?
- How might this trial affect my daily life?
- How long does the trial last?
- Will hospitalization be required?
- Who will pay for the treatment?
- Will I be reimbursed for other expenses, such as parking or bus fare?
- What type of long-term follow-up care is part of this study? Will I be able to receive the study medication after I have finished participating in the study?
- Will results of the trials be provided to me?
- Who will be in charge of my care?

Surgery Option

Although many patients, families, and physicians focus on medications as the primary means of treating IBD, drugs are just one aspect of the care of the patient. This care must encompass not only drug therapy, but must also address, where necessary, the nutritional and psychological aspects of the disease. In addition, surgery is a very important part of the management of IBD.

The need for surgery should not necessarily be considered a failure of the person with IBD, of his family, or of the health-care team. While recent advances in drug therapy may reduce the need for surgery in the future, surgery can provide patients in some situations with relief from symptoms that may not be possible using medications.

CHAPTER 8

Surgical Treatment of IBD

CASE STUDY Kelly

Kelly, the university student with ulcerative colitis, did very well with the drug treatment first prescribed by her specialist. She was put on prednisone and, although she did notice some swelling of her face and some weight gain, she was quite happy that her symptoms of abdominal cramps, diarrhea, urgency to move her bowels, and rectal bleeding subsided. Her prednisone dose was reduced over a period of 10 weeks and then stopped. She was placed on 5-ASA maintenance therapy to keep her well.

Although Kelly did well for 8 months, her symptoms came back with a vengeance during the following school year. Once again, she felt better with a 10-week course of prednisone, but experienced three more flares over the next 2 years, each one requiring a course of prednisone and each one improving less quickly and less completely than the flare before. The flares recurred despite being placed on the immunosuppressant drug azathioprine by a gastroenterologist, to prevent flares. Kelly even tried a number of naturopathic remedies and probiotic treatment out of desperation.

At her next appointment with her gastroenterologist, Kelly declares that she is "fed up" with her disease, with the medications, and with their side effects. She has missed several semesters of school because of her illness. She wants to get on with her life. Her gastroenterologist raises the possibility of surgery as a means of managing her disease. She knows that IBD can't be cured and wonders if surgery would be just a temporary fix. She wonders what type of surgery she would need. She also wonders if the surgery would leave her needing to have a bag to collect her stool. Will she be able to have children? She has heard that there are some newer surgical techniques that are less invasive and wonders whether she might be a candidate for one of those procedures. Her doctor was pleased to advise her on surgery options.

The Need for Surgery

Although there are many drug therapies for treating Crohn's disease and ulcerative colitis, there are cases where this treatment does not bring symptoms under adequate control or where the side effects of the treatment are too serious or are more than the patient can tolerate. The symptoms of IBD may be so severe, come on so suddenly, or persist for so long that surgery becomes a preferred or required treatment option. There are also cases where a complication of IBD may occur that cannot be addressed adequately with drug therapy but can be resolved with surgery.

Risk and Benefit Analysis

In some of these cases, the symptoms do not improve on treatment because the disease has resulted in damage or scarring of the intestine and medications typically do not reverse most forms of damage. As a result, the IBD sufferer may never feel entirely healthy and may have significant restrictions on work and social life despite being on medication. At that point,

Risk of Surgery

Approximately 70% to 80% of people suffering from Crohn's disease and approximately 20% to 40% of people suffering from ulcerative colitis will require surgery at some point following their diagnosis. These estimates are based upon information from previous decades and do not necessarily reflect the effect of recent advances in drug therapy. Nevertheless, there is still a substantial proportion of IBD sufferers who end up requiring surgery for their disease.

Q **What does surgery involve? How long will I need to stay in the hospital?**

A Most of the operations performed for IBD have certain features in common. First, the medical professional performing surgery will be a surgeon, usually someone other than the doctor who has been managing the other aspects of your treatment, typically a gastroenterologist (an internist with special training in treating gastrointestinal disorders). Second, most operations require one or more incisions on the abdomen in order for the surgeon to gain access to the involved areas of intestine. Third, most operations require a general anesthetic and a stay in hospital following surgery. The length of the hospital stay depends, to a large degree, on the nature of the operation, but averages somewhere around 7 to 10 days. Complications of surgery may increase the time in hospital. Finally, the time until full recovery averages 6 weeks, but this is highly dependent upon the type of operation, the patient's general health and nutritional state prior to surgery, and the patient's level of motivation.

surgery may help the person to feel healthier, with fewer restrictions on work, school, or leisure activities. Although surgery does involve some risk — both the risk that it may not be completely effective or the IBD may recur and the risk that it can result in a complication — and although surgery always involves some time away from work, school, or usual activities and always involves some degree of pain and discomfort, there comes a point where the suffering caused by the IBD is greater than these risks of surgery. Put another way, at some point an IBD sufferer decides to accept these real and potential risks of surgery in order to have a better chance of feeling well.

Ileostomy and Colostomy

One form of surgery for IBD is an ostomy — either an ileostomy or a colostomy. "Ostomy" is the generic term for a procedure that brings an opening in the intestine out through the layers of the abdominal wall and the skin. This is sometimes referred to as a stoma.

If the last part of the small intestine (ileum) is brought out to the skin, this procedure is specifically called an ileostomy, and if the large intestine (colon) is brought out to the skin, it is called a colostomy. In both procedures, either a cut end of the intestine or a loop of intestine is brought through the skin. Where a loop is brought out, it is usually a temporary ostomy with the intention to close it or, if necessary, convert it to a permanent end ostomy. With the end ostomy, the wall of the intestine is turned out after it is brought out through the abdominal wall and its edge is sewn to the surrounding skin.

A colostomy is usually flat or flush with the surrounding skin, while an ileostomy usually sticks out several centimeters above the level of the skin.

Because the stoma consists of the inner lining of the intestine, it is normally pink or red and may look painful or sore. However, the stoma has no pain-detecting nerve fibers and, as a result, is not actually painful to touch.

Because stomas do not have a valve or sphincter, there is no way to control if and when stool or gas is excreted from the stoma. As a result, a stoma requires an appliance or bag that fits over it to collect the stool and prevent soiling.

Some people delay or refuse to have surgery because they do not want to consider having an ileostomy. In some cases, this means that the person becomes sicker and sicker and more debilitated because their IBD is not adequately controlled by medications. When they finally do end up having surgery,

No Standard Procedure

There is no "standard surgery" for IBD; rather, there are a small number of operations that cover most of the situations. The exact nature of the surgery needs to be individualized in the same way that drug therapy must be individualized based upon a patient's particular circumstances, the area of the GI tract affected, and the objectives of the surgery.

they may be at increased risk of complications because they have become sicker and weaker and they may have reduced immunity against infections. As a result, the healing of surgical incisions may not be as good and they are at increased risk of infections. Fortunately, for most people, the idea of having an ileostomy is worse than the reality of having an ileostomy, particularly when having the surgery that results in an ileostomy has such a significant impact on one's sense of well-being. Once the diseased bowel is removed surgically, the person typically starts to feel better, their nutritional state begins to improve, and their immunity improves. Despite the fact that most patients adapt well to an ileostomy, it is still not what anyone would consider to be an "ideal" outcome, all other considerations aside.

Q **If I need surgery for IBD, does it mean that I'll need to wear a bag on my abdomen to collect my stool?**

A Surgery for IBD does not necessarily mean that you will have to wear a bag or appliance to collect stool from the stoma. In fact, most people undergoing surgery do not need to wear a bag after undergoing surgery or, if it is needed, it is most often temporary until the stoma is reversed or closed.

Surgical Procedures for Ulcerative Colitis

While the colectomy with an ileostomy was the most common operation in ulcerative colitis until the 1970s and 1980s, the ileostomy has been replaced in most cases with the pelvic pouch procedure.

Colectomy

When considering surgery, patients with ulcerative colitis have a major advantage over patients with Crohn's disease because their disease involves only the large intestine (colon): when the large intestine is surgically removed, the disease is effectively "cured."

Ileostomy, Colostomy, Diverting Loop Ileostomy

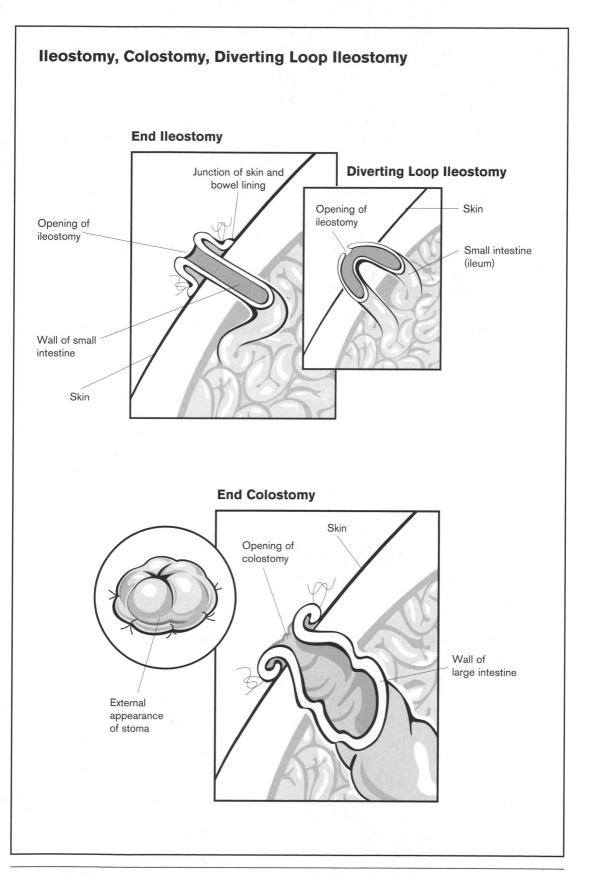

End Ileostomy

Junction of skin and bowel lining

Opening of ileostomy

Wall of small intestine

Skin

Diverting Loop Ileostomy

Opening of ileostomy

Skin

Small intestine (ileum)

End Colostomy

Skin

Opening of colostomy

Wall of large intestine

External appearance of stoma

Living with a Stoma

Most people who have a stoma do very well with it and are able to adapt as necessary. There is seldom a need to change everyday activities or avoid physical activity. Competitive sports and sexual relations are possible for someone who has had the procedure performed. Immediately after surgery, the stoma may be somewhat swollen, but this will usually go down during the first 6 weeks after surgery. A stoma should almost never get in the way of leading a full and active life.

Appliances

The apparatus that attaches to the skin and that holds the bag over a stoma is known as an appliance. Several types of appliances are available, each with its own advantages and disadvantages. Patients may have to try several different appliances before finding one that works well for their build, stoma location, and lifestyle.

The assistance of an enterostomal therapy nurse (ET nurse) can be extremely valuable in avoiding frustration and in finding an appropriate appliance as quickly as possible after surgery. The ET nurse can also play an important role in the education of the IBD sufferer about the proper care and maintenance of the stoma, thereby reducing the possibility of future problems.

Self-consciousness

People are often concerned about the appliance being obvious under clothing, but, in most instances, others will not be aware that you have a stoma unless you actually tell them. An enterostomal therapy nurse can help you with various methods or tricks to try to keep the appliance hidden.

Stool Consistency

The consistency of the stool coming out of the stoma varies depending on diet, fluid intake, and the time of day. There is a period of adaptation after surgery when the stool may go from being mainly liquid to having a thicker consistency. With an ileostomy, the stool generally gets to a consistency of porridge or toothpaste after several weeks or months, but it is almost never fully formed or solid. With a colostomy, the stool may eventually become solid.

Odor and Gas

Odor and gas are also concerns. Odor is usually not a problem as long as the appliance fits properly over the stoma and does not leak. An odor usually only occurs when the bag is emptied. This is generally done in a bathroom, and air fresheners can help mask the odor. Proper cleaning of the lower edge of the bag, where the stool is emptied from, will also help avoid odor once the bag has been emptied.

Gas may be a more difficult problem to deal with. Try to avoid air swallowing, mouth breathing, smoking, gum chewing, and drinking fizzy or carbonated drinks, which all tend to increase the amount of gas passing through the stoma into the appliance. If there is a lot of gas, it results in the bag filling up very quickly and requiring more frequent emptying.

Fluids and Electrolytes

Because patients with an ileostomy do not have a functioning colon, their ability to absorb water and electrolytes may be diminished. This is normally not a problem, but people who are chronically dehydrated may be at higher risk of certain types of kidney stones. In hot weather, when someone with an ileostomy may have increased loss of fluid and electrolytes from sweat, be sure to maintain an adequate water intake (at least 2 to 3 quarts/L per day) and to take plenty of salt with your food — or, if necessary, take salt tablets.

Intimate Relationships

Before starting sexual activity, it is important not to have a full appliance. Some people prefer to use special smaller appliances and straps or devices, which secure the appliance during sexual activity. Once again, your enterostomal therapy nurse can help you to find the right appliance for your needs. You may also find that certain activities or positions are more satisfying or more secure for you and your partner. This requires a certain amount of experimentation or trial and error.

Entering into a new sexual relationship can pose particular challenges for someone with a stoma. Although your partner may not even be aware that you have a stoma during the time that you first become acquainted, it is generally a good idea to be honest and open about the stoma before going down the path of sexual intimacy. This can be a very critical time in a relationship, usually requiring a certain degree of stability.

> ### Disclosure
>
> A stoma does not have to interfere with intimacy and sexual relations with a spouse or partner, but there is no question that it does require the understanding of the spouse or partner and often some time to adjust. You may feel "dirty" or "undesirable" on account of the stoma. Telling your partner about your concerns and fears is an important step. Your partner may also have concerns or questions that you can help answer.

The nature of the explanation that you give to your partner needs to be tailored to both of your needs, but it should usually include an indication that you had surgery for an intestinal problem and that the surgery has allowed you to recover your health to the point where you feel well enough to be sexually intimate. Your partner should also understand that, as a result of the surgery, part of your intestine has been brought out through the skin and that you have to collect the stool in a secure bag or appliance.

Removing the large intestine is called a colectomy. Because the rectum is always diseased in ulcerative colitis, it has to be removed along with the rest of the large intestine; as a result, it is not possible to reattach the lower end of the small intestine to any part of the large intestine.

Before the late 1970s and early 1980s, undergoing a colectomy meant that the small intestine had to be brought through an incision in the skin as an ileostomy so that the fecal waste material would drain into an external appliance or bag. For most people with ulcerative colitis, that was the end of their problems with inflammatory bowel disease. They were able to discontinue all medications, and they felt healthy without experiencing bleeding or abdominal pain.

However, the operation left them physically changed. For many individuals, the idea of a permanent ileostomy was not easy to accept. Despite the fact that most patients adapt well to an ileostomy, it is still not what anyone would consider to be an "ideal" outcome, all other considerations aside.

Pelvic Pouch Procedure

To address the adverse personal reactions that may occur to the usual ileostomy, surgeons have developed the pelvic pouch procedure, also known as the ileal pouch anal anastomosis (IPAA). This procedure is now offered to most patients who require a colectomy for ulcerative colitis. Patients over the age of 60 and those with damage to the anal sphincter (valve) mechanism, primarily women who have experienced damage to the sphincter during a difficult or traumatic childbirth, may not be candidates for the operation. The large majority of ulcerative colitis patients who undergo the pelvic pouch procedure are pleased with the results of the operation.

In the pelvic pouch procedure, the colon and most of the rectum are removed. Then the surgeon takes the lower end of the small intestine (ileum), partially opens it up, and folds it back upon itself to fashion it into a large-capacity pouch. The pouch is then attached to the remaining very bottom part of the rectum, which is just above the anus.

In most situations, the small intestine above the pouch is brought out to the skin as a temporary ileostomy, which is reversed (closed) in a second operation 3 to 6 months later. The temporary ileostomy effectively prevents the fecal material from going through the pouch in order to allow it to heal well or, at least, to reduce the negative consequences and risk of infection if there is a problem with healing.

When a patient is very sick, poorly nourished, or on high doses of steroids at the time the colectomy is performed, the

High Satisfaction

The pelvic pouch procedure is offered to most patients who need surgery for ulcerative colitis. More than 90% end up being very satisfied with the result.

Gas

Although gas is not necessarily a sign of a problem with the pouch, it can be embarrassing, and the larger amounts of gas production can also cause patients to feel that they have to move their bowels more frequently than they normally would.

Pelvic (Ileal) Pouch Procedure

Panel 1

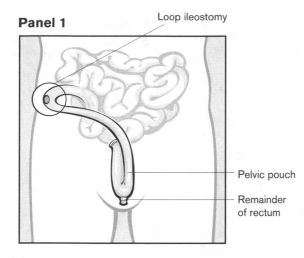

Loop ileostomy

Pelvic pouch

Remainder of rectum

The pelvic pouch procedure is usually done in two or three stages. Initially, the pouch is formed by folding the small intestine (ileum) back on itself to make a "J" shape. The bottom of the "J" is opened and sewn to the small segment of remaining rectum (detail panel). The temporary loop ileostomy is created above the pouch (panel 1), and several months later the ileostomy is closed (panel 2), thus producing an intact digestive tract (panel 3).

Panel 2

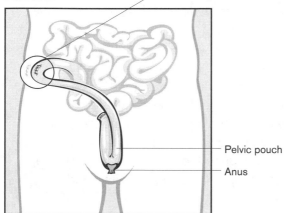

Closed ileostomy

Pelvic pouch

Anus

Detail Panel

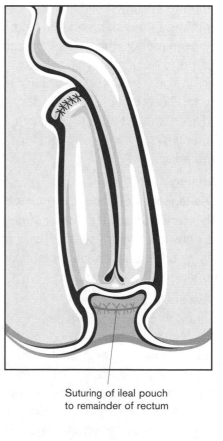

Suturing of ileal pouch to remainder of rectum

Panel 3

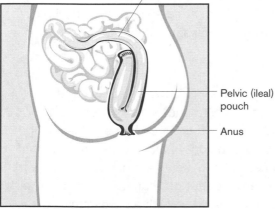

Small intestine above the pouch

Pelvic (ileal) pouch

Anus

Living with a Pelvic Pouch

Following pelvic pouch surgery and closing of the temporary ileostomy, patients usually take several weeks or months to become accustomed to the functioning of the pouch.

Bowel Movements

Patients will typically have anywhere from 4 to 12 bowel motions per day, but usually without cramps, urgency, or bleeding. The average number of bowel motions is 6 to 8 per day. The stool often has a soft or loose consistency, but may be somewhat formed in some patients. However, frequency of bowel motions can vary widely, depending on many factors, including how much fluid is being consumed and the types of food in the diet.

Stool Odor and Consistency

Many patients who have had the pelvic pouch procedure report changes in the smell of the stool and in the amount and smell of gas. The stool tends to be very irritating to the skin, and if it is not cleaned off well after a bowel motion, the skin can become red, itchy, painful, or even break down. Barrier creams containing zinc can sometimes be helpful in protecting the skin.

In some instances, the consistency of the stool and smell of the gas can be modified by adjusting the diet. Although there are certain foods that are advised against in individuals who have undergone the pelvic pouch procedure, finding foods that agree and don't agree with you is usually a matter of trial and error.

Soiling

Leakage of stool from the anus can occur following the pelvic pouch procedure. This tends to occur primarily during sleep; it is usually a minor amount leading to only some minor soiling. This can usually be managed by putting a small pad inside one's underwear or nightclothes. Regular episodes of loss of stool control during the daytime are rare.

Bowel Control

Although patients with a pelvic pouch may have more bowel motions than would be considered "normal" and the stool is often looser and perhaps even smellier than normal, the fact that they can usually control their need to move their bowels, that they no longer need medications to control their symptoms, and that they feel well offsets these inconveniences. Most patients are quite satisfied with the procedure; they are generally far and away better off than they were prior to surgery and better off than they imagine they would be with an ileostomy.

Very Loose Stools

For people with very loose or watery stools, supplementation of the diet with a source of soluble fiber, such as psyllium, may be helpful. For some individuals, antidiarrheal medications, such as loperamide (Imodium), can reduce the frequency of bowel motions enough to make them much more comfortable, particularly in social or work situations.

---

creation of the pouch is usually delayed until the patient is in better health, better nourished, and off steroids.

Complications

A number of complications of the pelvic pouch procedure can occur. Some of these are related to the operation itself — the risk of a general anesthetic, pneumonia, blood clot in the legs or lungs, and wound infection or wound opening — and go along with any type of abdominal surgery. Some of these complications are relatively minor and can be managed, but others can pose serious obstacles to patients who want to return to a normal life and good health.

Bowel Obstruction

Perhaps the most common complication is a bowel obstruction or blockage, which results in abdominal pain, nausea, vomiting, and usually a decrease in bowel motions. This can occur as soon as several days or a week following surgery and is thought to be due to adhesions (scar tissue) that form on the outside of the intestine after surgery. These adhesions can lead to kinking or twisting of the bowel, causing obstruction.

Infections

In the pelvic pouch procedure, the suturing (stitching) or stapling where the pouch is created or attached to the rectum can leak or come apart. This can lead to an abscess or serious infection in the abdominal cavity. Most pouch leaks will heal without having to operate again. However, it is important to avoid this type of complication before it occurs, because not only is it potentially serious in the short term, it also tends to lead to poorer functioning of the pouch months or years later once the leak has healed. This means that there may be more bowel motions on average, more potential leakage of stool, and possible problems with emptying the pouch.

Pouchitis

Another complication that can occur after pelvic pouch surgery is an inflammation of the inner lining of the pouch called pouchitis. This condition occurs in approximately 10% to 15% of patients undergoing the pouch procedure, although some centers that have a large experience with the pelvic pouch procedure report higher rates of pouchitis.

Pouchitis presents with symptoms of increased stool frequency and stool looseness, abdominal cramping, loss of control of bowel motions, blood in the stool, and not feeling well.

Obstruction Outcomes

Bowel obstructions that occur soon after surgery usually settle down on their own after several days, but they can cause increased pain and discomfort for the patient and can lengthen the stay in hospital. If the obstruction does not settle on its own, it may require surgery to relieve it. Some individuals can also develop obstruction months or years after the pelvic pouch procedure.

"Colitis" of the Pouch

Acute pouchitis occurs in 10% to 15% of people undergoing the pelvic pouch procedure. In many ways, it looks and feels like ulcerative colitis of the pouch.

Treating Pouchitis

Antibiotics: Bacteria are apparently important in causing pouchitis because it almost always responds to a 7- to 14-day course of antibiotics. This is quite different from ulcerative colitis, where antibiotics are not effective treatment. Ciprofloxacin (Cipro) is the antibiotic of choice for first treatment of pouchitis, but many doctors prescribe metronidazole (Flagyl) or a combination of the two.

A small percentage of patients who recover from a first episode of pouchitis develop repeated episodes. Usually, these respond again to another course of antibiotics, but some of these patients end up having some degree of ongoing or persisting pouchitis and may require regular antibiotic treatment to keep the pouchitis under some degree of control.

Probiotics: Another approach to controlling chronic pouchitis or preventing recurrent episodes is the use of probiotics, the so-called good bacteria, such as *Lactobacillus acidophilus* and bifidobacterium, which are normally present in the human intestine. When probiotics are taken, usually in the form of a capsule or as a powder mixed with food or drink, they may have a beneficial effect on the health of the pouch by preventing recurrent episodes of pouchitis. Probiotics may also be found in some types of yogurts.

Medications: When antibiotics are not helping someone with chronic pouchitis, some of the medications that are routinely used to treat ulcerative colitis are occasionally tried. These medications are often not very helpful.

Surgery: It is rare for a patient to require surgical removal of the pelvic pouch because of chronic pouchitis and poor pouch function. In those cases, an ileostomy is usually required because there is a high chance that if a new pouch is created, similar problems will occur again.

Surgical Procedures for Crohn's Disease

Unlike ulcerative colitis, Crohn's disease can affect any part of the gastrointestinal tract and can recur in previously unaffected segments of intestine following surgical resection of a diseased area. Although there are theoretically many different types of operations that can be performed for Crohn's disease, in practice a handful of operations account for the majority actually performed, chiefly small intestine and large intestine resections and perianal procedures.

The tendency for Crohn's disease to come back in previously unaffected segments of bowel is one of the main reasons that patients give for not wanting to undergo surgery for Crohn's disease. They worry that, after going to all of the trouble and taking on the pain and risk of surgery, they might be back at "square one" within a year or two of having undergone surgery. However, similar to the situation with ulcerative colitis, avoidance of surgery or excessive delays in going for surgery when the disease is not being adequately controlled by medications can result in progressive worsening of the patient's general status and reduced immunity. When surgery is finally carried out, this can lead to increased infections and complications and slower recovery times.

Small Intestinal Resection

The most common operation performed for Crohn's disease is a small intestinal resection. This is usually performed because an area of small intestine is affected by Crohn's disease, and this has led to scarring and narrowing of the intestinal opening through which food passes. This produces symptoms of pain, bloating, nausea, and vomiting after meals and can even lead to bowel obstruction. Small intestinal resections may also be required when a fistula or an abscess has arisen from an affected segment of intestine or when symptoms of active inflammation in the small intestine (abdominal cramping, diarrhea, weight loss) do not respond to drug therapies.

Ileocecal Resection

When the large intestine has no obvious Crohn's disease, only the very first part of the colon, called the cecum, is resected. This is called an ileocecal resection: the last part of the ileum and the first part of the colon are taken out together as a single piece of intestine.

> **Recurrence**
>
> Whereas removal of the large intestine in ulcerative colitis leads to a "cure" with no chance of ulcerative colitis recurring in the small intestine or other parts of the gastrointestinal tract, Crohn's disease can recur in previously unaffected segments of intestine following surgical resection of a diseased area. This may lead to the need for multiple operations and removal of additional intestinal segments at each operation.

Q **What is short bowel syndrome?**

A The surgical approach to Crohn's disease may require several different procedures and several repetitions of the same procedure. Ultimately, this can result in the removal of so much intestine that it leaves patients unable to keep themselves nourished and to maintain fluid and electrolyte balance through the intake of food and liquids. This condition, called short bowel syndrome, is a serious consequence of Crohn's disease surgery and can lead to the need for long-term or permanent intravenous feeding at home (home total parenteral nutrition, or HTPN).

To avoid this, there is a tendency, where it is safe, to delay surgery for Crohn's disease, and when surgery is needed, the surgeon will usually try to resect only the minimum amount of bowel necessary to deal with the immediate problem.

Extent of Resection

Although any part of the small intestine can be affected with Crohn's disease, the most common section is the last part of the small intestine (terminal ileum) just before the small intestine joins the large intestine. Because the diseased bowel and associated narrowing usually extends right up to the junction between the small and large intestine (ileocecal valve), it is technically impossible for the surgeon to remove just the small intestine, making it necessary to remove the ileocecal valve and an adjacent portion of the large intestine. The amount of large intestine resected is determined by whether or not it too is affected.

Ileocolic Resection

If part of the large intestine is affected by Crohn's disease — most commonly on the right side in an area involving the cecum and part of the ascending colon — then it is often resected along with the terminal ileum. This operation is called an ileocolic resection.

Small Intestinal Resection

When there is a normal segment of small intestine between the lowermost extent of the affected small intestine and the ileocecal valve, it is technically possible to remove only the affected segment of small intestine and not remove any of the large intestine. This is called a small intestinal resection.

Anastomosis

In all of these operations, the removal of a segment of intestine leaves two unattached, or open, ends of small intestine or one open end of small intestine and one of large intestine. These ends are sewn or stapled together to re-establish the continuous flow of intestinal contents all the way through the gastrointestinal tract.

However, in some situations, the surgeon may decide to create a temporary stoma above the surgical hookup site (anastomosis) in order to divert the intestinal contents away from the anastomosis so that it has the best chance of healing fully. This is usually done when there has been an abscess or uncontrolled infection in the area of the anastomosis prior to surgery and the risk of poor healing is higher. In most cases, the stoma is closed during another surgical procedure several months later.

Strictureplasty

Patients who have had multiple previous intestinal resections or who have multiple segments of affected small intestine are at risk of developing short bowel syndrome if they have more of their bowel removed surgically. A strictureplasty is a method of avoiding removal of additional segments of intestine. There are a number of methods of performing strictureplasty, but they all involve opening up the affected and narrowed segment of the

Strictureplasty

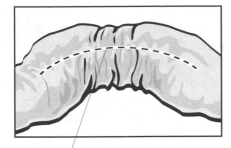

Narrowed section

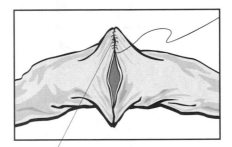

Incision

The narrow segment of the intestine has an incision made along its length and is then sewn across to widen the opening.

Sewn together

Seton

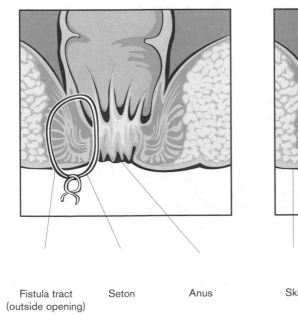

Fistula tract (outside opening)   Seton   Anus

Abscess Drainage

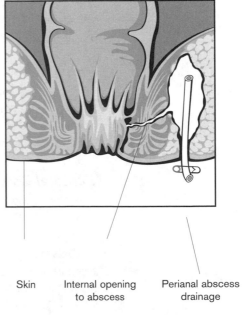

Skin   Internal opening to abscess   Perianal abscess drainage

intestine and creating a larger internal passageway for food to pass through without causing symptoms of obstruction.

Strictureplasty is not always done whenever there is a narrowed segment of small intestine, for several reasons. The affected segment is often too long — multiple short segments of narrowing are ideal for strictureplasty. The segment is sometimes too diseased and thickened, making it difficult to work with surgically. There may be only a single short segment of narrowing, and the risk of the strictureplasty procedure (leak, infection, recurrent obstruction) is not worth the potential benefit of avoiding a resection, which is generally much easier to perform. In the situation where the affected segment is very short, then resection of that segment carries very little risk of complication or of future development of short bowel syndrome.

Large Intestinal Resection (Colectomy)

Removal of all or part of the large intestine is less commonly done in Crohn's disease than is a small intestinal resection. It is typically performed when all or part of the colon is affected with Crohn's disease and the symptoms cannot be controlled with medication. Occasionally, the operation is performed because of one or more strictures in the colon or because of a fistula or abscess arising out of the colon.

There are a few common segments of colon that may be removed, and each of these operations has its own name describing the part of the colon that has been removed: the right half of the colon in a right hemicolectomy, the left half of the colon in a left hemicolectomy, and the sigmoid colon in a sigmoid resection.

Partial Colectomy

When a colectomy is performed, it may be partial or complete. In a partial colectomy, only a portion of the large intestine is removed and usually the two cut ends of the intestine are sewn together.

Subtotal Colectomy

A subtotal colectomy involves removal of all of the large intestine, with the exception of the rectum and perhaps the lower end of the sigmoid colon. In this operation, the last part of the small intestine (ileum) is connected to the rectum to form an ileorectal anastomosis or to the sigmoid colon to form an ileosigmoid anastomosis.

Pelvic Pouch Option

Most surgeons who perform the pelvic pouch procedure will offer the operation to a patient who appears to have ulcerative colitis, but in whom Crohn's disease cannot be absolutely ruled out, as long as there are no abscesses, fistulas, or ulcers in or around the anus, there is no evidence of a problem with function of the anal sphincter, and the patient understands that there is a higher risk of pouch failure.

Total Proctocolectomy

If the entire colon and rectum are removed, the operation is called a total proctocolectomy. The end of the small intestine is usually brought out to the skin as an ileostomy. Patients with known Crohn's disease are usually not candidates for pelvic pouch reconstruction surgery, except in special circumstances.

Pelvic Pouch Surgery

Ulcerative colitis does not recur once the rectum and colon have been removed, but Crohn's disease can come back in the pouch and in the small intestine above the pouch if the patient has undergone the pelvic pouch surgery. This frequently leads to poor pouch function, medical complications, and a very unhappy patient who has gone through several operations with the expectation of being "cured."

Only in Select Circumstances

If someone has Crohn's disease involving the rectum and colon, the pelvic pouch procedure is usually not offered as an option, except in very select circumstances.

Mistaken Ulcerative Colitis

Although pelvic pouch procedures are, in most circumstances, not offered to patients with known Crohn's disease, there are some patients who, despite extensive examination and investigation prior to surgery, are thought to have ulcerative colitis but subsequently are discovered to have Crohn's disease. This can occur once the entire colon has been removed and examined under a microscope by a pathologist or after being followed for many years after surgery and found ultimately to develop features of Crohn's disease, such as ulcers in the small intestine above the pouch.

In these cases, the patient with Crohn's disease is left with a pelvic pouch. Antibiotics, steroids, immunosuppressants, and especially infliximab have been found to be quite helpful in this setting, although the experience is still rather limited. A significant proportion of patients with Crohn's disease and a pelvic pouch — somewhere around 1 in 4 — will end up requiring further surgery and very possibly surgical removal of the pouch, with the creation of a permanent ileostomy.

Small and Large Intestine Resection

Small intestine resection

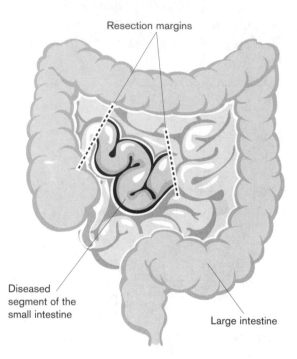

Resection margins

Diseased
segment of the
small intestine

Large intestine

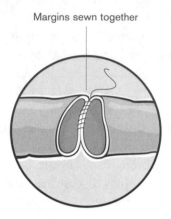

Margins sewn together

When a resection is performed,
the diseased segment of intestine
is cut out and the remaining margins are sewn together.

Large intestine resection

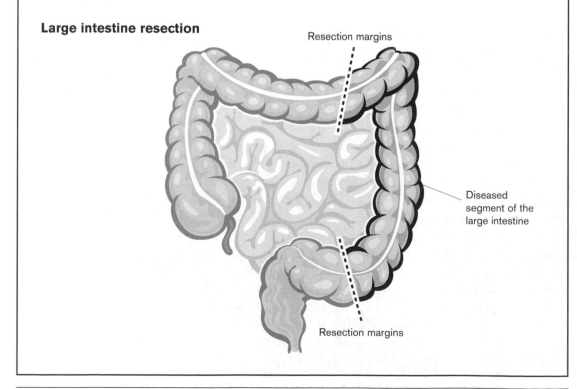

Resection margins

Diseased
segment of the
large intestine

Resection margins

Mapping Fistulas and Abscesses

Many operations for perianal Crohn's disease are preceded by investigations to help map out where the fistulas, if present, communicate with the rectum or with each other and to look for any abscesses that may be present but not suspected by the usual examination that can be performed in the clinic.

Physical Examinations and Tests

The usual examination involves visually inspecting the area around the anus, feeling the area around the anus, and using a finger to feel inside the anus and rectum. Other investigations include CT scan, MRI, and endoanal ultrasound. Endoanal ultrasound involves putting an ultrasound probe into the anus and rectum. The probe emits a high-frequency sound wave that bounces off the tissues and back to the probe. These sound waves are detected by the probe and converted into images on a screen. Which investigation is performed really depends on what is available at a given center and the expertise of the doctors performing the tests.

Surgical Examination

The surgery for perianal disease almost always involves an examination by the surgeon once the patient has been put under a general anesthetic (examination under anesthesia). The muscles in the area are all relaxed once the patient has received a general anesthetic, and this allows a better examination with probing of the fistula openings. The examination under anesthesia may actually help map out the disease as well as, or in some cases better than, the tests discussed above.

Indeterminate Colitis

In some cases when IBD involves only the colon, Crohn's disease cannot be differentiated from ulcerative colitis, even when the entire colon has been removed and examined by a pathologist. In that situation, called indeterminate colitis, the pelvic pouch procedure may be offered to patients with the understanding that some will ultimately turn out to have Crohn's disease, with a higher chance of failure of the pouch procedure. However, when all patients with indeterminate colitis undergoing the pelvic pouch procedure are compared to patients with ulcerative colitis, patients with indeterminate colitis have only a slightly higher risk of pouch failure.

Perianal Surgeries

Unlike the surgery for treatment of Crohn's disease involving the intestine, surgery for the complications of Crohn's disease in the area of the anus (perianal disease) does not usually involve removing any segments of bowel.

Most operations are performed to reduce the symptoms of the perianal disease — most often pain and drainage of pus or stool — when the symptoms have not responded to other measures, such as sitz baths, antibiotics, immunosuppressants, and infliximab or adalimumab, or when an acute problem, such as an abscess, has occurred.

Incision and Drainage

Once the surgeon has adequately mapped out the extent of abscesses or fistulas, a procedure is chosen to reduce or eliminate the patient's symptoms. In some cases, this may involve cutting open the skin near the anus in order to allow an abscess to drain (incision and drainage).

Fistulotomy

In other cases, where there is a single fistula that does not cut across the anal sphincter, the surgeon may open up the fistula with an incision along its length (fistulotomy). This, in turn, allows the fistula to heal from the inside out, thereby eliminating the fistula tract.

Seton

Where there are multiple fistulas or when the fistula crosses the anal sphincter, this type of fistulotomy is not possible because of the likelihood of causing damage to the sphincter, which would result in problems with loss of control of the bowels (incontinence).

Instead, the surgeon may pass a string, thread, or thin plastic band through the outside opening of the fistula on the skin around the anus, along the fistula tract as it passes under the skin and toward the anus or rectum, through the internal opening of the fistula inside the anus or rectum, and back out through the anal canal. The two ends of the string are tied together, effectively creating a loop through the fistula and the anus. This string or tube, also known as a seton, keeps the fistula open and allows it to drain in a controlled way.

This result would seem to be the opposite of one of the objectives of treating perianal disease — that is, reducing drainage from the fistula. However, in many patients with fistulas, the openings of the fistulas periodically close up, thereby causing the pus that normally drains out to collect inside. This, in turn, causes more inflammation in the tissues around the fistula and the anus, and an abscess can form. Anyone who has ever had a perianal abscess knows that it is exquisitely painful and can interfere with simple activities, such

---

Seton Option

For a person who keeps developing recurrent abscesses, a seton is a preferable option. Although it may be associated with some local irritation and drainage, it is usually minor compared to the pain that can occur when an abscess forms.

---

as sitting, walking, and sleeping. It can also become acutely painful during a bowel motion.

The abscess must then be drained by a surgeon or, in many instances, will go away once the fistula tract has opened again on its own. Recurrent inflammation in the perianal area can lead to scarring and damage, thus making it more difficult for the area to eventually heal.

Surgical Flap

Occasionally, surgeons may attempt to repair or close off the internal opening of a fistula where it comes through inside the anus or rectum. This is most often tried when the fistula connects the rectum and the vagina. The surgical procedure involves taking a flap of tissue that is partially cut out of the inner lining of the rectum and pulling it down and over the opening of the fistula that exists inside the rectum. The flap is sewn over the opening in an attempt to keep it in place. Other methods of closing fistulas have been tried. One of these involves injecting a substance that forms a gel-like plug into the outside opening of the fistula. There have been some reports of good results with this technique, but it cannot be considered a standard practice until more experience has accumulated and better results have been demonstrated.

Failure Rate

Surgical flap operations, which, under the best of circumstances, have a fairly high failure rate of approximately 40% to 50%, should only be attempted if the rectum is free of active Crohn's disease and should only be performed by a surgeon experienced in the management of Crohn's disease fistulas.

Combined Approach

An approach that is often used to manage perianal Crohn's disease is a combined surgical and medical approach, whereby the surgeon drains any abscesses and puts in setons as necessary and the gastroenterologist treats the Crohn's disease with medication, most often infliximab or adalimumab. Although there haven't been large trials to study this combined approach, it appears that it may provide long-term healing and symptom control better than what can be provided by either surgery or drug therapy alone.

In addition, if a patient has active intestinal disease with resulting diarrhea, this will tend to aggravate the symptoms of the perianal disease. If drug treatment is effective in healing the intestinal lining and reducing diarrhea, this alone will have a noticeable and beneficial effect on the perianal disease.

Unfortunately, this type of combined approach is not readily available everywhere because in some areas the surgeons and gastroenterologists may not work closely together or they may not have the necessary expertise and experience in dealing with this complicated form of Crohn's disease.

Diverting Loop (Temporary) Ileostomy

For patients with severe perianal fistulas who do not respond to these measures or who have had damage to the anal sphincter, a diverting loop (temporary) ileostomy may be the operation that provides them with the best outcome.

By preventing stool from passing through the anus and the area of the fistulas and abscesses, this particular operation may result in a reduction in drainage from the fistulas, reduced abscess formation, and, in some cases, healing of the fistulas or surgical wounds left behind after drainage of an abscess. In those instances, the ileostomy may be reversed, or closed, and the fistulas will sometimes, but not always, remain healed.

End Ileostomy

For the patients with anal sphincter damage, closure of the ileostomy may not be feasible because incontinence will occur or the fistulas and abscesses may recur. In these cases, the loop ileostomy may be converted to a more permanent end ileostomy once the affected individual becomes accustomed to having a stoma. This type of ileostomy usually functions somewhat better than the temporary type and is easier for the individual to care for.

Removal of Rectum

When the rectum is left behind and not used for many years, there appears to be risk of cancer of the rectum. This can be difficult or impossible to screen for, and diagnosis usually occurs late and after the chance for cure has passed. As a result, most surgeons and gastroenterologists recommend that the rectum be removed electively before cancer has had a chance to develop. This is best done once the patient's nutritional state has improved and stabilized and once the patient is off medications, such as prednisone.

Reducing Cancer Risk

If patients have had an end ileostomy for the treatment of rectal and perianal disease, it is usually recommended that they eventually have the rectum and anus removed surgically and the area closed up to reduce the risk of cancer of the rectum.

Laparoscopic Surgery

Since approximately 1990, laparoscopic surgery has been used for many different types of gastrointestinal disorders, such as gallbladder disease and appendicitis. This type of surgery, sometimes referred to as "minimal access surgery" or "keyhole surgery," involves using instruments that are passed through several (usually three or four) small incisions on the abdomen. One of the instruments is a camera that allows the surgeon to see inside the abdomen without opening it up with a large

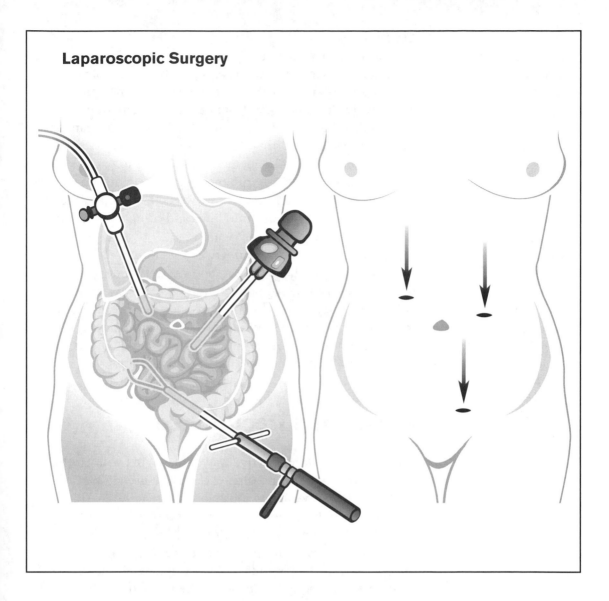

Laparoscopic Surgery

incision. The other instruments act as the "hands" of the surgeon, used for cutting, suturing, stapling, and all of the other things that a surgeon would normally do during a standard open-approach operation.

When a piece of an organ, such as the intestine, is removed, the incision at the belly button is usually extended a few centimeters to allow the intestine to be brought out. The advantage of the laparoscopic approach is that it leaves very small scars on the abdomen. These are often not noticeable unless one closely examines the area. In addition, it appears to reduce, to some extent, but does not eliminate the pain after surgery and allows faster discharge from hospital. For some operations, such as gallbladder, it allows quicker recovery and return to work or school.

Limitations

Even when a laparoscopic approach is planned when an operation is started, it is not always possible to complete the entire operation this way because there may be many adhesions (scars) within the abdomen from previous surgery that make it impossible to see well enough using the laparoscopic camera. In other cases, the Crohn's disease is too complex, with many internal fistulas from one segment of intestine to another or an abscess associated with an inflamed segment of intestine. Using a laparoscopic approach in this case would be unsafe. When surgeons encounter these limitations and complications, they will convert to an open approach.

Although laparoscopic surgery can result in major reductions in pain, hospital stay, and recovery time, these benefits over the open approach in the average case of IBD are not as obvious. There is still post-operative pain requiring medication, a hospital stay that averages about 5 days if no complications occur, and 3 to 6 weeks before someone is ready to return to work, school, and other daily activities.

Preventing Recurrence

Surgery can be a very effective way of managing your Crohn's disease. However, Crohn's disease can come back in parts of the intestine that were previously not affected. As a result, it is not unheard of for people with Crohn's disease to require two, three, four, or even more operations.

If you have had multiple operations and if a large part of your intestine has been taken out, you may ultimately not be able to adequately absorb nutrients, water, minerals, and electrolytes from your diet. This can be a very serious problem — more serious than the Crohn's disease itself. At the end of the day, the real challenge in the field of surgery for Crohn's disease is not so much how to perform an operation, but how to prevent the disease from coming back after the diseased bowel has been removed.

Recurrence Risk

Approximately, 1 out of every 3 patients undergoing surgery for Crohn's disease will have a recurrence of symptoms within 3 to 5 years if they are on no treatment, and a portion of those will end up requiring another operation.

However, it appears that some individuals are at lower risk of recurrent Crohn's disease and may not need treatment after surgery. Unfortunately, there is no good way to predict who is at high risk and who is at relatively low risk.

Stop Smoking

Perhaps the best way to reduce the risk of recurrence of Crohn's disease after surgery is not to smoke cigarettes. Although it has not been proven that for smokers who quit after surgery the risk of recurrent disease is lower, it has been shown that smokers tend to have earlier and more severe recurrences after surgery. So, if you don't already smoke, don't start after surgery, and if you do smoke, consider attempting to quit. Not only will this benefit your Crohn's disease, but it will have other health benefits (reduced heart disease, lower cancer risk, less lung disease).

Medications

Some patients, particularly those who have had a very short segment of intestine removed or who had disease for many years before coming to surgery, may choose not to take medication following surgery. For some patients, one goal in undergoing surgery is to stop medication, and this needs to be considered in discussing the management of Crohn's disease after surgery.

Although the 5-ASA medications are probably the safest and best tolerated, they have a very modest effect on the risk of recurrence, reducing the risk of recurrence by about 10% to 12%. Metronidazole and other related antibiotics also appear to reduce recurrence, but not all patients are able to tolerate the medications because of a metallic taste in the mouth and gastrointestinal upset. It is not clear whether the beneficial effect of antibiotics extends past 1 year after surgery.

The immunosuppressants azathioprine and 6-mercaptopurine are being used more often for prevention of recurrence after surgery for Crohn's disease, despite the fact that the evidence supporting their use is not entirely clear. Nevertheless, there is a sense among expert IBD physicians that these drugs are among the best maintenance treatments available and, if monitored properly, have good safety records. These drugs are used particularly when a person has had very severe or complicated disease prior to surgery, if a relatively long length of intestine has been surgically removed, or if it is not the first operation for Crohn's disease.

Infliximab has been shown to be effective for the treatment of acute flares of Crohn's disease as well as maintenance therapy. Because of its effectiveness in those situations, there has also been interest in using infliximab after surgery. There is some evidence that it is an effective preventive treatment after surgery, but it still remains to be determined which patients would benefit most from its use.

Follow-up Colonoscopy and Medications

In an effort to determine which patients to recommend for preventive treatment after surgery, particularly for treatment

> **Drug Effectiveness**
>
> A number of different medications have been tried as a way to reduce the risk of recurrent Crohn's disease after surgery. None of the currently available drugs are 100% effective. The ones most commonly used are 5-aminosalicylic acid (5-ASA) containing preparations, antibiotics, and azathioprine or 6-mercaptopurine (6-MP). These are all discussed in more detail in the chapter on drug therapy.

with an immunosuppressant drug, such as azathioprine or 6-mercaptopurine, or an anti-tumor necrosis factor drug, such as infliximab or adalimumab, some gastroenterologists are conducting a colonoscopy at some point in the first 12 months after surgery. It is well known that early signs seen by colonoscopy can occur well before symptoms of Crohn's disease recur, and this provides an opportunity to treat the Crohn's disease before the lesions progress to more severe types of lesions, which can then frequently result in symptoms and complications. Patients who develop these lesions within the first year after surgery are at higher risk for having more progressive or aggressive disease recurrence, and they are then offered the opportunity to go on drug therapy.

Q **Can I still become pregnant after surgery?**

A In general, women are still able to get pregnant after having had surgery for IBD. However, in some cases, when there has been a lot of inflammation and scarring in the area low down in the abdominal cavity and in the pelvis, where the ovaries and fallopian tubes sit, it may be more difficult for a woman to get pregnant.

Although most operations by themselves do not seem to result in problems conceiving, there is one procedure that may be somewhat different – the pelvic pouch procedure. It has recently been observed in several centers where the procedure is performed that women who have the pelvic pouch procedure for management of ulcerative colitis may be less able to get pregnant after the surgery. The exact proportion of women undergoing the procedure who cannot get pregnant is not known but may be as high as 1 out of every 3. This is different from the experience with the operation that used to be done for ulcerative colitis – the total colectomy with a permanent ileostomy – where the ability to get pregnant did not seem to be affected. It is not known why the pelvic pouch procedure might interfere with the ability to get pregnant, but it is thought to be due to the scarring that occurs around the fallopian tubes as a result of the operation. This prevents the eggs from the ovaries from getting into the uterus.

Children with IBD

These concerns about surgery, drug therapy, and recurrence of IBD are especially important when treating children with Crohn's disease and ulcerative colitis. Parents play a vital role in translating this complex information to their children, while helping them to make the "right" decision for treatment.

Q What drugs are safe for women who have IBD and become pregnant?

A None of the drugs that are used for IBD are known without a doubt to be safe in pregnancy because the types of studies needed to prove complete safety have not been done and are unlikely to ever be done. Despite this, there is a considerable amount of experience using most of the drugs, and there does not appear to be any evidence of increased risk to the pregnancy or to the fetus with most drugs used for IBD. The one definite exception is methotrexate, which has been definitively shown to cause spontaneous abortions and malformations of the fetus.

Because they are relatively newer, there is somewhat less experience using the anti-tumor necrosis factor drugs infliximab and adalimumab in pregnancy. However, in the time that they have been on the market, a substantial number of pregnant women have been treated with these drugs and there does not appear to be any increased risk of bad pregnancy outcomes or congenital malformations. The drug does pass through into the fetus in the last trimester of pregnancy and it can still be detectable for up to several months after birth. So far, this has not resulted in any reported side effects for the infants of mothers on infliximab or adalimumab, but it is generally recommended that infants not receive live vaccines during the first 6 months of life if their mothers were taking one of these two drugs in the last trimester of pregnancy. This transfer of drug from mother to baby has raised questions regarding whether infliximab or adalimumab should be temporarily stopped during the final months of pregnancy.

There is considerable controversy surrounding this issue and, although it appears that the drug might be able to be stopped for a few months at the end of pregnancy without a huge risk of IBD flare, the risk does seem to increase the longer the woman is off treatment. In addition, if anti-tumor necrosis factor therapy is restarted after a gap of several months, there may be an increased risk of subsequent allergic reactions and possibly reduced long-term effectiveness of the drug. These factors need to be considered by the woman and her doctor when deciding on what to do about therapy with infliximab or adalimumab in the later stages of pregnancy.

The other anti-tumor necrosis factor alpha drug, certolizumab pegol (Cimzia), does not appear to cross over to the baby's circulation during pregnancy and may provide some theoretical advantage over the other two drugs during pregnancy. However, in most instances where a pregnant woman is already taking infliximab or adalimumab during pregnancy and doing well from the perspective of her IBD, it is not advisable to switch medications.

CHAPTER 9

Treating Children with IBD

CASE STUDY Michael

Michael is a 14-year-old boy who has always been a good student. He has been popular and active in sports, especially hockey. Over the past year or so, he has experienced occasional episodes of abdominal pain and diarrhea. These have usually lasted only a few days, going away on their own. Although Michael missed a day or two of school and sports activities during these episodes, they did not occur often and his parents did not think much about them.

However, Michael noticed that most of the boys on his hockey team were getting much bigger and were going through puberty, whereas he had not experienced the growth spurt, deepening of the voice, and body hair growth that his friends had experienced. The size difference made it more difficult to compete in hockey. He was also feeling more tired than usual.

When he paid his annual visit to his pediatrician, Michael was routinely weighed and measured. His doctor pointed out that his rate of linear growth (height) had fallen off over the last 2 years. Previously, he was at the 50th percentile for his age — in other words, he had been just about average — but now he was at the 10th percentile, meaning that approximately 90% of boys his age are taller than him. The pediatrician was concerned with this growth delay, as well as Michael's fatigue and abdominal symptoms.

She decided to order some blood tests and an upper GI series and small bowel follow-through. These showed evidence of anemia and iron deficiency on blood testing — and an 8-inch (20 cm) segment of small intestine that looked like it was affected with Crohn's disease. She referred Michael to a pediatric gastroenterologist, who carried out a colonoscopy and then discussed the treatment options with Michael and his parents.

Available treatments included both drug treatment (steroids, immunosuppressives, infliximab), nutritional therapy, and surgery. After much discussion of the pros and cons, Michael and his parents elected to try nutritional therapy with feeding of a liquid nutritional supplement through a nasogastric tube and iron supplementation. Michael was taught to place the tube himself through his nose and into his stomach each evening and remove it each morning. During the daytime, he primarily took a fluid diet, but occasionally had some favorite food — french fries, potato chips, or other snack foods — when he was with his friends. After several months of therapy, Michael's energy level improved and he was not experiencing any more episodes of abdominal pain and diarrhea. His checkup at 3 months indicated that he had grown an inch (2.5 cm) and was showing some signs of entering puberty.

Family Challenges

Crohn's disease and ulcerative colitis are two chronic disorders that commonly affect children. If you are the parent of a child with IBD, you will know that the management of the disease in your child presents special challenges. The disease can cause great strain within the family unit, and even the strongest families may find it difficult to cope with the stress of having a child with a chronic illness for which there is no cure. This can be particularly difficult when children are very young and do not know what is happening to them. Trying to explain to children why they are not feeling well is never easy.

Parents may find it more difficult to cope with the symptoms, medications, hospitalizations, and prospect of possible surgery associated with their child's disease than the child does. For the most part, children tend to be very resilient and adapt well to new situations and new challenges, especially when given appropriate support. The support of parents, other family members, and the health-care team can help the child meet the challenges ahead. The support of friends and teachers is also important.

> ### Childhood Risk
>
> Approximately 20% of individuals with IBD develop the disease when they are children or adolescents. IBD is very uncommon in infants and toddlers, but the incidence gradually increases during childhood and adolescence

Special Management

Although Crohn's disease and ulcerative colitis in children are similar in many ways to IBD in adults, the way the disease presents and the way it is managed require special consideration.

Disease Type

When inflammatory bowel disease is recognized in very young children, under 5 years of age, the inflammation is usually in the colon. This colitis could be either chronic ulcerative colitis or Crohn's colitis. In very young children, the appearance of the disease in the colon is not as well defined as in teenagers and adults, making it harder to distinguish the type of colitis.

Outside of the preschool age group, the percentage of children and teenagers with Crohn's disease or ulcerative colitis is similar to the percentage observed among adults in the same geographic region. In North America, for example, Crohn's disease occurs more commonly than ulcerative colitis in adults and in older children and teenagers.

Intestinal Location

The locations of the disease in the intestinal tract are somewhat different in children than in adults, although there is a large degree of overlap. In children with ulcerative colitis, the disease most commonly involves the entire colon (pancolitis or extensive colitis), whereas, in adults, up to 50% of ulcerative colitis sufferers will have inflammation limited to the last part of the colon and rectum.

In children with Crohn's disease, just as in adults, different parts of the intestinal tract can be inflamed. Apart from the very youngest children, the percentage of children and adolescents with small intestine, large intestine, and combined small and large intestine involvement with Crohn's disease seem to be similar to that of adults. Involvement of the upper part of the small intestine (jejunum) is not common in children (occurs in less than 10%), but it may be more common in children than in adults.

Growth and Development

Chronic diseases in children may affect growth and development. Not only the disease itself but also the treatments can pose problems.

Disease Effects

Inflammatory bowel disease itself can have a very important negative effect on growth, even before the disease is diagnosed.

Catch Up

Although the inflammation associated with IBD can result in a reduced rate of growth, adequate treatment of the IBD, whether through the appropriate use of medications, nutritional supplements, or surgical treatment, can allow a child to have some degree of "catch-up" growth. The rate of growth increases to a rate above normal so that the child, in effect, catches up to a height close to what it was destined to be before IBD developed. The target height, of course, is generally reflected by the parents' heights.

However, there is only limited opportunity for catch-up growth. Once the child reaches a certain age — which varies from child to child — further catch-up growth is no longer possible and the child may not attain the maximum possible height. For example, girls usually finish growing in height within 2 years of their first menstrual period. Boys generally enter puberty and finish growing on average 2 years later than girls.

A child can experience poor growth for several years before Crohn's disease is recognized and treated.

A fall-off in growth rate that occurs before a child develops symptoms, such as abdominal pain or diarrhea, may be very puzzling for the pediatrician and parent. The reason may only become apparent once other symptoms develop and a diagnosis of IBD is made. This effect on growth is much more commonly seen in Crohn's disease than in ulcerative colitis. The reasons for the difference are not well understood.

Drug Side Effects

Historically, many of the treatments used in adults have also been used in children, sometimes without solid proof that these treatments are as effective in children as they are in adults. Not all drugs commonly used in adults are necessarily desirable to use in children because of their potential for side effects and the concerns about long-term safety or delayed effects that may be observed many years after the drug is taken.

Steroids

Steroid medications, such as prednisone, are very effective at reducing the intestinal inflammation in both Crohn's disease and ulcerative colitis, and, as a result, they can improve symptoms, such as abdominal pain, diarrhea, and rectal bleeding. However, in children, they also have the potential to reduce growth noticeably, if they are used for extended periods.

Immunosuppressants

In Crohn's disease, there has been an increasing tendency to use immunosuppressive medications, such as azathioprine, 6-mercaptopurine, or methotrexate, whenever a child requires steroids to bring their disease symptoms under control. When effective, these drugs will allow the child to taper off the steroid without relapsing and will reduce the need for further courses of steroids over a period of several years. This avoidance of steroids may be very important in allowing the child to grow normally and reach full height potential. There has also been increasing use of anti-tumor necrosis factor antibody therapies in place of steroids to treat children with IBD.

Delayed Puberty

A slowing of growth in height is usually associated with a delay in pubertal development as well. Keeping pace with the growth and development of one's friends can be very important to the self-esteem of a child with IBD. When a child's friends are growing rapidly and developing the physical characteristics

> **Steroid Care**
>
> Doctors who treat children with Crohn's disease and ulcerative colitis will prescribe steroid medications for a significant flare-up of IBD, but they are careful to avoid long-term use of steroids, recognizing that this would have negative effects on growth.

of a mature woman or man, the child with IBD may still have the stature and appearance of a younger child. This can make it very difficult for the children to fit in with their peers and, unfortunately, can make it more likely that they will become the target of teasing or even bullying. Physical appearance problems may be compounded by the effect of a medication, such as prednisone, which can cause delayed growth, weight gain, and rounding of the face.

Inflammatory Proteins

Growth delay and the associated delay in pubertal development result from a number of different but interrelated factors. The most important factors seem to be inflammatory proteins produced by the diseased bowel. These proteins can have many effects, including reduction of appetite and thus food intake, and interference with growth hormone pathways. Controlling the activity of the disease through the appropriate use of medications or surgery, avoiding certain medications, such as steroids, and maintaining good nutrition can help to optimize a child's growth.

Irregular Periods

Once a girl has reached puberty and menstrual cycles have started, it is not uncommon for her to experience irregular periods or even to have her period stop, particularly when she is experiencing a disease flare. Encourage your daughter to bring this issue to the attention of her doctor, because irregular or absent menstrual periods may interfere with her developing strong bones. This, in turn, may lead to an increased risk of osteoporosis later in life.

Long-Term Treatment

Both Crohn's disease and ulcerative colitis are chronic disorders that cannot be cured by medical or nutritional therapy. Although surgery can be "curative" for ulcerative colitis, it is not a perfect solution because of early and late complications.

For every drug developed for the treatment of IBD, there are concerns about the delayed or long-term consequences of being on the medication, particularly if it is used continuously and if it is used from an early age. These effects cannot always be predicted based upon our knowledge of how the drug works, and they may not be apparent for many years after the drug is available for general use. As a result, the use of any new medication for the treatment of IBD is likely to involve a certain amount of risk taking, particularly when used in children.

An area of specific concern in children is the use of immunosuppressive medications. Although this class of medications has a very good safety record, they do, as their name suggests, suppress the body's immune system to a certain extent and, as a result, can lead to a slightly increased risk of infections. In addition, there is some evidence to suggest that azathioprine and 6-mercaptopurine (6-MP) result in a slightly increased risk of lymphoma (cancer of the lymph glands).

This cancer is quite uncommon. Even for individuals taking azathioprine or 6-MP, the risk is still very small — probably somewhere in the range of 1 in 5,000 to 1 in 10,000. The risk does appear to be somewhat higher in young males, and there is one particularly aggressive form of lymphoma, heptosplenic T-cell lymphoma, that seems to occur almost exclusively in young males treated with azathioprine or 6-MP. Many IBD patients and their families are willing to accept these small potential risks, particularly if there is immediate benefit to be had by being on the medications.

Psychological Issues

For parents, it's tough enough raising a child without having to deal with a chronic illness such as IBD. The addition of IBD to the mix creates some special psychological challenges to the parent–child relationship.

Parenting Styles

Different parents have different ways of reacting to illness in a child. There is no absolute wrong or right way of interacting with a child with a chronic disease as long as a supportive and caring environment is maintained. IBD is a challenge that should be approached together as a family.

Growing Independence

Working with a child with IBD depends on the age of the child. In younger children, parents have to take a very active role in the monitoring and management of the disease. However, this should be done in a supportive way so as not to be intrusive or smothering. Children should have enough "room" to become independent over time, eventually taking an active role in managing their disease.

Team Approach

Taking a "team" approach with children, whereby they are given a certain degree of defined responsibility for monitoring and managing their disease, is frequently an effective parenting strategy. This responsibility may involve remembering to take medication at certain times or reporting back to the parent about any unusual symptoms.

Positive Parenting Attitudes

- Your child may have inflammatory bowel disease, but this does not mean that you love or value your child any less.
- Your child is not at fault for having developed IBD.
- You are not at fault for your child having developed IBD.
- Your child has not disappointed you.

Positive Reinforcement

Positive reinforcement through encouragement and by providing small inexpensive rewards, such as stickers, can be helpful in keeping the child interested and active in disease management. Ultimately, you hope your child takes on these roles without these rewards by realizing that being proactive works well in management of the disease.

Adolescence

The relationship between a parent and a child changes considerably, and may become more challenging in the face of a chronic disorder, as the child enters adolescence. In adolescence, the importance of family relationships may diminish while the importance of friends and peers increases. When adolescents have IBD, the natural tendency of parents to be closely involved in their care may fly in the face of their desire to become more independent. This can be a source of tension between parent and child.

The adolescent may use the management of the disease as a means of asserting independence, sometimes with negative effects when, for example, asserting one's independence means not taking prescribed medications (or not telling parents whether the medication has been taken), not being open about symptoms, and not attending appointments with doctors. There is no easy solution to this problem, but when it occurs, these acts of rebellion tend to be part of a larger pattern of independent behavior. Approaching the overall situation rather than specifically focusing on the disease and its management may be an effective way of improving cooperation.

Adolescents may also become angry and frustrated with the disease — the symptoms, the examinations, the medications, and the occasional hospitalizations. Just when they are trying to be like their friends, the disease reminds them that they are, in some ways, different. In addition, the flares of disease and the associated symptoms may get in the way of their ability to attend school regularly and to take part in typical adolescent social and leisure time activities — sports, parties, dating, or just hanging out with friends. Although it may sometimes be difficult to connect with an adolescent, parents, teachers, and friends can all help at these trying times.

Prospects

During the past few decades, inflammatory bowel disease has become more familiar to primary care physicians and pediatricians. As a result, a diagnosis of IBD is usually made early on and is reasonably accurate by using a combination of investigations, such as blood tests, imaging studies, endoscopy, and biopsies.

Although there is no cure for Crohn's disease or ulcerative colitis, once the diagnosis has been made, nutritional counseling, psychological support, drug therapy, and surgery can all help in the right circumstances.

Research continues into the causes of IBD, and breakthroughs, such as the identification of the first Crohn's disease susceptibility gene, provide hope that the causes will be identified and that preventive strategies can be employed in individuals at risk of developing IBD. In addition, the development of new biologic therapies that are founded on advances in research into the altered immune response hold out the hope for newer, more effective therapies over the coming years.

In the meantime, close cooperation between the IBD sufferer and the health-care team provides the best opportunity for effective management of these chronic diseases. This book offers a foundation for that cooperation by providing patients, families, and health-care providers with practical information to assist them in making informed recommendations and decisions.

Realistic Expectations

Be sure to set realistic expectations about the course of the disease, since even with the best management and adherence to medications, disease flares and hospitalizations can occur. This should not be viewed as a failure of either the parents or the child.

Resources and References

Associations and Agencies

Atlas of Inflammatory Bowel Disease
www.endoatlas.com/atlas_ib.html
Features pictures taken during colonoscopy or gastroscopy of areas of the gastrointestinal tract affected by Crohn's disease and ulcerative colitis.

Gastrointestinal Society:
Canadian Society of Intestinal Research
855 West 12th Avenue, Vancouver, BC V5Z 1M9
Tel: 1-866-600-4875 (toll free in Canada)
E-mail: info@badgut.org
www.badgut.org
A registered charity that works to increase awareness, provides free educational materials to patients and health professionals, and funds medical research in the area of digestive diseases and disorders.

ClinicalTrials.gov
www.clinicaltrials.gov/ct/search?term=inflammatory+bowel+disease
Features the U.S. National Institutes of Health list of all registered clinical trials in inflammatory bowel disease in the United States, Canada, and elsewhere.

Cochrane Collaboration
www.cochrane.org
The Cochrane Collaboration is an organization dedicated to collecting and synthesizing all of the available research data on a wide variety of health-care interventions so that evidence-based recommendations for treatment can be made.

Crohn's and Colitis Foundation of America
386 Park Ave S, 17th Floor, New York, NY 10016
Tel: 800-932-2423
E-mail: info@ccfa.org
www.ccfa.org
This foundation supports research in inflammatory bowel disease and also provides educational support for patients and families.

Crohn's and Colitis Foundation of Canada
600-60 St. Clair Ave E, Toronto, ON M4T 1N5
Tel: 1-800-387-1479
www.ccfa.ca
This patient-founded organization is dedicated to finding the cure for IBD and features an online forum for "Frequently Asked Questions" and "Ask the Doctor" questions.

Food and Drug Administration Center for Food Safety and Applied Nutrition
www.fda.gov/AboutFDA/CentersOffices/OfficeofFoods/CFSAN/default.htm
An excellent American resource on food safety and labeling, as well as links to several useful publications.

Health Canada — Food & Nutrition
www.hc-sc.gc.ca/fn-an/index-eng.php
An excellent Canadian resource on food safety and labeling, as well as links to several useful publications.

Mount Sinai Hospital Inflammatory Bowel Disease Group
600 University Ave, Toronto, ON M5G 1X5
www.zanecohencentre.com/ibd
The multidisciplinary Mount Sinai Hospital IBD Group in Toronto provides information for patients, health-care providers, and researchers, including two videos — one on life after a stoma and the other on the pelvic pouch procedure.

National Digestive Diseases Information Clearinghouse
2 Information Way, Bethesda, MD 20892–3570
Tel: 1-800-891-5389 Fax: 703-738-4929
E-mail: nddic@info.niddk.nih.gov
www.digestive.niddk.nih.gov
Information dissemination service with general information about various digestive diseases, including Crohn's disease and ulcerative colitis.

Ontario Human Rights Commission — Employment: Your Rights and Responsibilities
www.ohrc.on.ca/en/issues/employment
This site describes your rights as a prospective employee in the province of Ontario, which may be applicable to other jurisdictions in North America.

United Ostomy Associations of America
PO Box 512, Northfield, MN 55057-0512
Tel: 800-826-0826
E-mail: info@ostomy.org
www.ostomy.org
This network for bowel diversion support groups in the United States benefits people who have had intestinal diversions and their caregivers. It also includes groups for people who have had urinary diversion procedures.

United Ostomy Association of Canada
344 Bloor St W, Suite 501, Toronto, ON M5S 3A7
Tel: 1-888-969-9698
www.ostomycanada.ca
This volunteer-based organization provides emotional support, as well as instructional and information services, to individuals who have had intestinal diversion procedures and to their caregivers.

Resource Books for Patients

If This Is a Test, Have I Passed Yet?
Living with Inflammatory Bowel Disease
by Ferne Sherkin-Langer (Fern Publications, 1994)
This is a friendly and useful firsthand account of what it is like to live with IBD and some strategies that proved to be useful.

Learning Sickness: A Year with Crohn's Disease
By James M. Lang (Capital Books, 2005)
This is an account of a year in the life of a man who finally has to come to accept that his Crohn's disease is a part of his life that requires special care.

Sick and Tired of Feeling Sick and Tired:
Living with Invisible Chronic Illness
By Paul J. Donoghue and Mary E. Siegel (W.W. Norton, 2000)
A more thorough overview of the issues of living with an invisible illness by two psychologists.

Codeine Diary:
True Confessions of a Reckless Hemophiliac
By Tom Andrews (Harvest Books, 1999)
This is not a book about IBD, but about living with hemophilia. Still, it is a very well-written account of many experiences living with a chronic recurrent disease that will be familiar to those with Crohn's disease or ulcerative colitis.

**Always Change a Losing Game:
Playing at Life to Be the Best You Can Be**
By David Posen (Firefly Books, 1997)
Includes several sensible approaches to stress reduction.

The Feeling Good Handbook
By David D. Burns (Plume, 1999)
This well-written self-help book introduces the techniques of cognitive-behavioral therapy for depression and includes homework exercises.

Full Catastrophe Living: Using the Wisdom of your Body and Mind to Face Stress, Pain, and Illness
By Jon Kabat-Zinn (Delta, 1990)
Meditation techniques for stress reduction and health.

Medical Texts and Journal Articles

Ardizzone S, Maconi G, Sampietro GM, Russo A, Radice E, Colombo E et al. Azathioprine and mesalamine for prevention of relapse after conservative surgery for Crohn's disease. Gastroenterology 2004;127(3):730-40.

Candy S, Wright J, Gerber M, Adams G, Gerig M, Goodman R. A controlled double blind study of azathioprine in the management of Crohn's disease. Gut 1995;37(5):674-78.

Casillas S, Delaney CP. Laparoscopic surgery for inflammatory bowel disease. Dig Surg 2005;22(3):135-42.

Duchmann R, Kaiser I, Hermann E, Mayet W, Ewe K, Meyer zum Buschenfelde KH. Tolerance exists towards resident intestinal flora but is broken in active inflammatory bowel disease (IBD). Clin Exp Immunol 1995;102(3):448-55.

Ekbom A, Helmick C, Zack M, Adami HO. Ulcerative colitis and colorectal cancer. A population-based study. N Engl J Med 1990;323(18):1228-33.

Elson CO, Cong Y. Understanding immune-microbial homeostasis in intestine. Immunol Res 2002;26(1-3):87-94.

Farmer RG, Whelan G, Fazio VW. Long-term follow-up of patients with Crohn's disease. Relationship between the clinical pattern and prognosis. Gastroenterology 1985;88:1818-25.

Feagan BG. Maintenance therapy for inflammatory bowel disease. Am J Gastroenterol 2003;98(Suppl 12):S6-S17.

Feagan BG, Rochon J, Fedorak RN, Irvine EJ, Wild G, Sutherland L et al. Methotrexate for the treatment of Crohn's disease. The North American Crohn's Study Group Investigators. N Engl J Med 1995;332(5):292-97.

Fefferman DS, Farrell RJ. Endoscopy in inflammatory bowel disease: Indications, surveillance, and use in clinical practice. Clin Gastroenterol Hepatol 2005;3(1):11-24.

Geboes K, De Hertogh G. Indeterminate colitis. Inflamm Bowel Dis 2003;9(5):324-31.

Gillen CD, Walmsley RS, Prior P, Andrews HA, Allan RN. Ulcerative colitis and Crohn's disease: a comparison of the colorectal cancer risk in extensive colitis. Gut 1994;35(11):1590-92.

Gionchetti P, Rizzello F, Helwig U, Venturi A, Lammers KM, Brigidi P et al. Prophylaxis of pouchitis onset with probiotic therapy: A double-blind, placebo-controlled trial. Gastroenterology 2003;124(5):1202-09.

Greenberg GR, Feagan BG, Martin F, Sutherland LR, Thomson AB, Williams CN et al. Oral budesonide for active Crohn's disease. Canadian Inflammatory Bowel Disease Study Group. N Engl J Med 1994;331(13):836-41.

Griffiths AM, Ohlsson A, Sherman PM, Sutherland LR. Meta-analysis of enteral nutrition as a primary treatment of active Crohn's disease. Gastroenterology 1995;108(4):1056-67.

Hanauer SB, Feagan BG, Lichtenstein GR, Mayer LF, Schreiber S, Colombel JF et al. Maintenance infliximab for Crohn's disease: The ACCENT I randomised trial. Lancet 2002;359(9317):1541-49.

Jarnerot G, Hertervig E, Friis-Liby I, Blomquist L, Karlen P, Granno C et al. Infliximab as rescue therapy in severe to moderately severe ulcerative colitis: A randomized, placebo-controlled study. Gastroenterology 2005;128(7):1805-11.

Johnson GJ, Cosnes J, Mansfield JC. Review article: Smoking cessation as primary therapy to modify the course of Crohn's disease. Aliment Pharmacol Ther 2005;21(8):921-31.

Kornbluth A, Legnani P, Lewis BS. Video capsule endoscopy in inflammatory bowel disease: Past, present, and future. Inflamm Bowel Dis 2004;10(3):278-85.

Kruis W. Review article: Antibiotics and probiotics in inflammatory bowel disease. Aliment Pharmacol Ther 2004;20 (Suppl 4):75-78.

Lofberg R, Danielsson A, Salde L. Oral budesonide in active Crohn's disease. Aliment Pharmacol Ther 1993;7(6):611-16.

Loftus EVJ, Silverstein MD, Sandborn WJ, Tremaine WJ, Harmsen WS, Zinsmeister AR. Crohn's disease in Olmsted County, Minnesota, 1940-1993: Incidence, prevalence, and survival. Gastroenterology 1998;114(6):1161-68.

Markowitz J, Grancher K, Kohn N, Lesser M, Daum F. A multicenter trial of 6-mercaptopurine and prednisone in children with newly diagnosed Crohn's disease. Gastroenterology 2000;119(4):895-902.

Maunder RG. Evidence that stress contributes to inflammatory bowel disease: Evaluation, synthesis, and future directions. Inflamm Bowel Dis 2005;11(6):600-08.

Mawdsley JE, Rampton DS. Psychological stress in IBD: New insights into pathogenic and therapeutic implications. Gut 2005; 54(10):1481-91.

McDonald JWD, Burroughs AK, Feagan BG (eds.). Evidence-based Gastroenterology and Hepatology, 2nd edition. Oxford, UK: Blackwell Publishing, 2004.

McLeod RS. Surgery for inflammatory bowel diseases. Dig Dis 2003;21(2):168-79.

Munkholm P, Langholz E, Davidsen M, Binder V. Frequency of glucocorticoid resistance and dependency in Crohn's disease. Gut 1994;35(3):360-62.

Rutgeerts P, Van Assche G, Vermeire S, D'Haens G, Baert F, Noman M et al. Ornidazole for prophylaxis of postoperative Crohn's disease recurrence: A randomized, double-blind, placebo-controlled trial. Gastroenterology 2005;128(4):856-61.

Sands BE, Anderson FH, Bernstein CN, Chey WY, Feagan BG, Fedorak RN et al. Infliximab maintenance therapy for fistulizing Crohn's disease. N Engl J Med 2004;350(9):876-85.

Sartor RB, Sandborn W (eds.). Kirsner's Inflammatory Bowel Diseases, 6th edition. Philadelphia, PA: WB Saunders, 2004. Satsangi J, Sutherland LR. (eds.) Inflammatory Bowel Diseases. Philadelphia, PA: Elsevier Limited, 2004.

Shen B, Fazio VW, Remzi FH, Lashner BA. Clinical approach to diseases of ileal pouch-anal anastomosis. Am J Gastroenterol 2005;100(12):2796-2807.

Sutherland LR, Martin F, Bailey RJ, Fedorak RN, Poleski M, Dallaire C et al. A randomized, placebo-controlled, double-blind trial of mesalamine in the maintenance of remission of Crohn's disease. The Canadian Mesalamine for Remission of Crohn's Disease Study Group. Gastroenterology 1997;112(4):1069-77.

Sutherland LR, May GR, Shaffer EA. Sulfasalazine revisited: A meta-analysis of 5-aminosalicylic acid in the treatment of ulcerative colitis. Ann Intern Med 1993;118:540-49.

Library and Archives Canada Cataloguing in Publication

Steinhart, Allan Hillary, 1959-
 Crohn's & colitis : understanding & managing IBD / A. Hillary Steinhart. — 2nd ed.

Includes index.
ISBN 978-0-7788-0401-7

 1. Crohn's disease. 2. Ulcerative colitis. I. Title. II. Title: Crohn's and colitis.

RC862.E52S74 2012   616.3'44   C2011-907461-3

Index

C

caffeine, 121, 123
calcium, 111
  sources, 106–9
  supplementation needs, 166, 167
calories, 111
Canada's Food Guide to Healthy Eating,
  96–97, 100, 112
cancer
  IBD and, 32–33
  medication as cause, 175, 219
CARD 15 gene, 81
Carnation Breakfast Anytime, 115
CAT/CT (computer-assisted tomography)
  scans, 48
certolizumab pegol (Cimzia), 183, 213
childbirth, 68–69. *See also* pregnancy
children
  bone density in, 31–32
  breast-fed, 77
  Crohn's disease symptoms, 39
  diagnostic tests for, 45, 50
  education concerns, 61–62
  growth concerns, 216–17
  medications for, 172, 173, 217,
    218–19
  parenting, 219–20
  psychological factors, 219, 220
  treatment for, 214–20
  and tube feeding, 126
cholangitis, primary sclerosing (PSC), 30,
  33
cholestyramine (Questran), 111, 121
Cimzia (certolizumab pegol), 183, 213
ciprofloxacin
  for Crohn's disease, 148, 170,
    171–72
  for pouchitis, 198
  during pregnancy, 68, 171–72
Clostridium difficile, 75, 172
codeine phosphate, 121
Colazide (balsalazide), 159–60
colectomy, 190, 194, 202–3
colitis. *See also* ulcerative colitis
  Clostridium difficile as cause, 172
  indeterminate (IBDU), 23, 205

colon (large intestine), 12, 18. *See also*
  colonoscopy; colostomy
  removal of, 190, 194, 202–3
colonoscopy, 12, 32, 50–53
  after surgery, 211–12
colostomy, 65, 189–90. *See also* stoma
communication
  with doctors, 40–41, 145–47, 152–53
  with family and friends, 142–43
Cortenema, 169
Cortifoam, 169
Crohn's disease, 10–11. *See also*
  inflammatory bowel disease
  case studies, 34, 72, 90, 132, 148,
    214
  medications, 148, 154, 170–73, 179,
    180
  nutritional therapy, 115
  perianal, 207
  recurrence prevention, 210–12
  smoking and, 14, 67, 210–11
  support resources, 143–44
  surgical procedures, 198–208
  symptoms, 22–23, 39, 42–43
cyclosporine, 168, 177–79
cytokines, 38

D

dairy products, 104, 107, 120. *See also*
  lactose intolerance
dehydration, 123, 193
depression, 135–38, 140
  medications for, 135, 137
  steroids as cause, 166
  symptoms, 136, 137
diabetes, 166
diarrhea, 38, 43
  medications for, 70, 121
  traveler's, 69, 70
diclofenac. *See* NSAIDs
diet, 90–131. *See also* nutrition
  advice sources, 91–92, 96–99, 131
  elimination, 101–2
  fiber in, 116–19, 120
  fluids as, 122–25
  fluids in, 71, 193

glucagon, 131
glutamine, 131
granulomas, 13, 23
guarana, 121

H

herbal products, 113–14
hospitalization, 64, 188
Humira (adalimumab), 29–30, 180, 183, 213
Hycort (hydrocortisone), 169
hydration, 123, 193. *See also* fluids
hydrocortisone, 169
hydrogen breath test, 103–4
hygiene, 78
hypertension, 166

I

ibandronate, 167
IBD. *See* inflammatory bowel disease
IBS (irritable bowel syndrome), 11, 13
ileostomy, 65, 189–90, 208. *See also* stoma
  after colectomy, 203
  and fluid intake, 193
  and lactose intolerance, 105
  temporary, 194, 208
ileum, 13. *See also* ileostomy; pelvic
  pouch procedure
  ileal brake, 121
  removal of, 199
imaging studies, 47–50
immune system, 17, 21. *See also*
  immunosuppressants; inflammation;
  lymphocytes
  gene mutations and, 81
immunonutrition, 128–30
immunosuppressants, 172–79
  after surgery, 211
  for children, 217, 218–19
  and infection, 85–86, 151, 174, 178
  side effects, 151, 173–75, 217
Imodium, 70, 121
Imuram (azathioprine), 172–76, 219
incontinence (fecal), 12, 20, 37, 196
  and travel, 70

infection
  biologic drugs and, 182
  as IBD cause, 74–76
  immunosuppressants and, 85–86, 151, 174, 178
  as pelvic pouch complication, 197
infertility, 67
inflammation. *See also* immune system
  in gastrointestinal tract, 22–23
  in joints, 28
  omega-3 fats and, 128–30
inflammatory bowel disease (IBD), 10–11, 13. *See also* Crohn's disease; ulcerative colitis
  age at onset, 14
  causes, 72–87, 92
  complications, 23–33, 48
  coping strategies, 138–44
  diagnosis of, 44–54
  dietary strategies, 90–131
  as disability, 62, 63–64
  disclosing, 63, 193
  drug therapy for, 87, 168, 170–72
  environmental factors, 15, 76–79, 86–87
  extra-intestinal manifestations, 28–33, 43
  flares of, 35, 59–60, 68, 150–51
  gender and, 14
  genetic factors, 79–87
  geographic distribution, 14–15, 77
  infection and, 74–76
  onset, 14, 44, 59, 60
  prognosis, 55, 58–61, 221
  progress, 58–61
  psychological factors, 78, 133, 219, 220
  risk factors, 59, 82–83, 84
  support sources, 142–44, 147
  surgery for, 187–212
  symptoms, 34–44, 60
  of undetermined type (IBDU), 23
infliximab (Remicade), 179–82
  after surgery, 211
  for Crohn's disease, 173, 179
  and pregnancy, 213
  as rescue therapy, 168
  for skin lesions, 29–30

Internet
  information sources on, 222–25
  as support source, 143–44
interpersonal style, 138–40, 142–43
intestines. *See* colon; small intestine
inulin, 128
iron, 111
irritable bowel syndrome (IBS), 11, 13

J

Japan, 15, 77
jaundice, 30
jejunum, 13
Jews, 15
jobs, 62–64
Johne's disease, 75
joints, 28, 167
juices, 117, 123

K

kidneys, 178–79

L

lactose intolerance, 102–5, 106
Lee, Robert Mason, 144
lesions
  skin, 29–30
  skip, 22
L-form bacteria, 75
lifestyle changes, 65–67
liver, 20, 30
  medication damage to, 174, 177
Lomotil, 70, 121
lymphocytes, 13, 21

M

malnutrition, 93–95. *See also* nutrition
MCTs (medium-chain triglycerides),
  115
measles, 76
medications, 148–86. *See also* antibiotics;
  immunosuppressants; steroids; *specific
  medications and conditions*

adapted, 149
antidepressant, 135, 137
antidiarrheal, 70, 121
biologic, 179–84
as cancer cause, 175, 219
for children, 172, 173, 217
considerations, 148–53
dosage levels, 150
as flare cause, 150–51
information sources, 152–53
intravenous, 177, 179
liver damage from, 174, 177
NSAIDs, 79, 154
options for, 153–54
patient history of, 41
and pregnancy, 68, 168, 171–72, 173,
  213
for severe attacks, 168
side effects, 29, 31, 85–86, 150–52, 167,
  217
standard, 149–50, 155
traveling with, 71
menstrual cycle, 67, 218
6-mercaptopurine (Purinethol), 172–76,
  219. *See also* immunosuppressants
mesalamine (5-ASA) medications,
  156–62
after surgery, 211
benefits, 158
controlled-release, 157–59
as enemas, 160–62
during pregnancy, 68
as suppositories, 160, 161, 162
methotrexate, 176–77
during pregnancy, 68, 213
metronidazole (Flagyl), 170, 171
for pouchitis, 198
microparticles, 130
mineral supplements, 106–9, 110–14
monitors, 141
mood swings, 166
motility, 13
mouth, 17
MRI (magnetic resonance imaging), 49
mucosa, 13, 18
multivitamins, 112, 113
mycobacteria, 75

R

rashes, 29–30
rectum, 13, 20, 36–37
    bleeding from, 36
    inflammation of (proctitis), 22, 162
    removal of, 203, 208
relationships, 138–40. *See also* sexual
    activity
research studies, 73
    of diet, 91
    of nutrition, 127–31
    participating in, 184–85
    of twins, 76–77, 79
risedronate, 167

S

sacroiliitis, 28
Salofalk (5-ASA), 157
Scandishake, 115
school, 61–62
self-reliance, 139, 140
serosa, 13, 23
seton, 206–7
sexual activity, 27, 193
short bowel syndrome, 199, 200
side effects, 29, 31, 85–86, 150–52, 167,
    217. *See also* medications
    blood tests for, 151, 174–75, 178–79
skin problems, 29–30
skip lesions, 22
sleep problems, 66, 166
small intestine, 18, 199–200. *See also*
    duodenum; ileum; jejunum
smoking, 14, 66–67, 79, 210–11
sodium, 111, 124
soiling, 196. *See also* incontinence
sphincters (anal), 12, 21
steroids (glucocorticoid medications),
    162–70
    dependency on, 163, 164
    dietary supplements needed, 110,
    111
    and disease flares, 58–59
    as enemas, 169–70
    intravenous, 168

oral, 163–68
and osteoporosis, 31, 167
during pregnancy, 68, 168
as rescue therapy, 168
side effects, 164–68, 169–70, 217
as suppositories, 169–70
stoma, 65, 189, 190. *See also* colostomy;
    ileostomy
    living with, 192–93
    supplies for, 71, 192
    temporary, 200
stomach, 17–18
stools, 119–21. *See also* bowel
    movements; stoma
    blood in, 36
    consistency, 119–21, 192, 196
    leakage of, 196
    odor, 192, 196
    testing, 46
stress, 66, 78, 134–35
    assessing, 141
    coping with, 135
strictures, 13, 25–26. *See also* bowel
    obstruction
    and diet, 25
    dietary fiber and, 117
    surgery for, 26, 200–202
    symptoms, 42
sugars (in diet), 120, 123
sulfasalazine (5-ASA), 156–57
sulindac. *See* NSAIDs
supplements (nutritional), 106,
    107–9, 112–16. *See also specific
    nutrients*
    for Crohn's disease, 115
    enzymes as, 106
    herbal, 113–14
    liquid, 114–16
    minerals as, 106–9, 110–14
    regulation of, 113–14
    with steroid use, 110, 111
    tips for taking, 116
    vitamins as, 109–13
support-seeking style, 139–40, 142–43
suppositories
    mesalamine (5-ASA), 160, 161, 162
    steroid, 169–70

surgery, 64–65, 187–212. *See also specific procedures*
  colonoscopy after, 211–12
  for Crohn's disease, 198–208
  hospitalization after, 188
  laparoscopic, 208–10
  medications after, 211
  need for, 188
  and pregnancy, 67, 212
  risks, 188–89
  for strictures, 26, 200–202
  for ulcerative colitis, 190–98
synbiotics, 127–28

T

teenagers. *See* adolescents
TEN (total enteral nutrition), 126
tests
  blood, 45–46, 151
  for children, 45, 50
  genetic, 84–86
  lactose intolerance, 103–4
  for side effect potential, 151
  stool, 46
  white blood cell, 49–50
TPMT (thiopurine methyl transferase), 86, 175
TPN (total paraenteral nutrition), 126–27
  at home (HTPN), 199
travel, 69–71
treatment. *See also* medications; surgery; *specific treatments*
  for children, 214–20
  for depression, 135, 137–38
  diet as, 78
  for malnutrition, 94
  nutritional supplements as, 115, 125–27
  unnecessary, 85

trophic factors, 131
tube feeding, 126
tuberculosis, 75, 182
twin studies, 76–77, 79
Tylenol (acetaminophen), 154

U

ulcerative colitis. *See also* inflammatory bowel disease
  case studies, 10, 56, 132, 187
  medications for, 153–54
  smoking and, 14, 67
  surgical procedures for, 190–98
  symptoms, 22, 35–38
ulcers, 13
  bowel, 17
  skin, 29–30
ultrasound, 48, 205
USDA MyPlate Food Guidance System, 98, 100, 112

V

vaginal infections, 172
Vegetarian Food Guide Rainbow, 99, 100
villi, 13, 18
viruses, 76
vitamins
  multivitamins, 112, 113
  as supplements, 110–14
  vitamin B_{12}, 111, 112
  vitamin D, 109–10, 111

W

weight gain, 165
weight loss, 38, 43, 94. *See also* malnutrition

white blood cells, 13, 21
   tests for, 49–50
wireless capsule (PillCam) endoscopy, 53
work, 62–64

X

x-rays, 47–48, 49–50

Y

yeast infections, 172
yogurt, 128

Z

zoledronate, 167

More Great Books
from Robert Rose

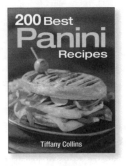

Appliance Cooking

- 200 Best Pressure Cooker Recipes
  by Cinda Chavich
- 200 Best Panini Recipes
  by Tiffany Collins
- The Juicing Bible, Second Edition
  by Pat Crocker
- The Mixer Bible, Second Edition
  by Meredith Deeds and Carla Snyder
- The 150 Best Slow Cooker Recipes, Second Edition
  by Judith Finlayson
- 650 Best Food Processor Recipes
  by George Geary & Judith Finlayson
- 125 Best Vegetarian Slow Cooker Recipes
  by Judith Finlayson
- Slow Cooker Comfort Food
  by Judith Finlayson
- The Dehydrator Bible
  by Jennifer MacKenzie, Jay Nutt & Don Mercer
- 300 Slow Cooker Favorites
  by Donna-Marie Pye
- 300 Best Bread Machine Baking Recipes
  by Donna Washburn and Heather Butt
- 300 Best Canadian Bread Machine Baking Recipes
  by Donna Washburn and Heather Butt

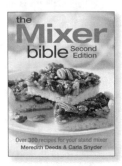

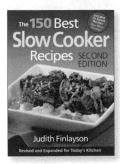

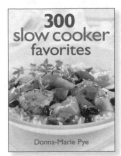

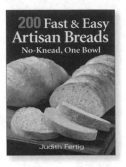

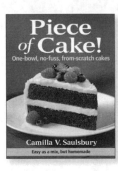

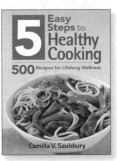

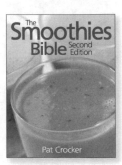

Baking

- Bake Something Great!
  by Jill Snider
- 200 Fast & Easy Artisan Breads
  by Judith Fertig
- 175 Best Babycakes Cupcake Maker Recipes
  by Kathy Moore & Roxanne Wyss
- 175 Best Babycakes Cake Pops Recipes
  by Kathy Moore & Roxanne Wyss
- 150 Best Cupcake Recipes
  by Julie Hasson
- Piece of Cake!
  by Camilla V. Saulsbury
- 750 Best Muffin Recipes
  by Camilla V. Saulsbury
- Complete Cake Mix Magic
  by Jill Snider

Healthy Cooking

- 5 Easy Steps to Healthy Cooking
  by Camilla V. Saulsbury
- 125 Best Vegan Recipes
  by Maxine Effenson Chuck and Beth Gurney
- The Vegetarian Cook's Bible
  by Pat Crocker
- The Vegan Cook's Bible
  by Pat Crocker
- The Smoothies Bible, Second Edition
  by Pat Crocker

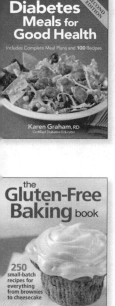

- Diabetes Meals for Good Health, Second Edition
  by Karen Graham, RD
- Canada's Diabetes Meals for Good Health
  by Karen Graham, RD
- 200 Best Lactose-Free Recipes
  by Jan Main
- 500 Best Healthy Recipes
  Edited by Lynn Roblin, RD

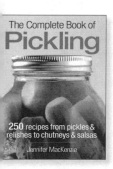

- The Gluten-Free Baking Book
  by Donna Washburn and Heather Butt
- Complete Gluten-Free Cookbook
  by Donna Washburn and Heather Butt
- 250 Gluten-Free Favorites
  by Donna Washburn and Heather Butt
- 250 Essential Diabetes Recipes
  Edited by Sharon Zeiler, BSc, MBA, RD
- Canada's 250 Essential Diabetes Recipes
  Edited by Sharon Zeiler, BSc, MBA, RD

Recent Bestsellers

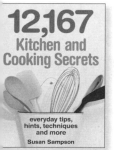

- The Complete Book of Pickling
  by Jennifer MacKenzie
- 12,167 Kitchen and Cooking Secrets
  by Susan Sampson
- 200 Easy Homemade Cheese Recipes
  by Debra Amrein-Boyes

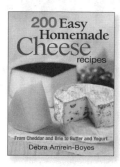

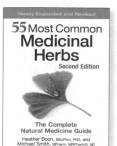

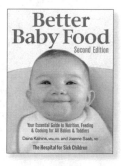

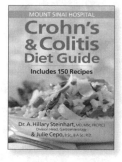

- Baby Blender Food
  by Nicole Young
- 750 Best Appetizers
  by Judith Finlayson and Jordan Wagman
- Simply Thai Cooking, Third Edition
  by Wandee Young & Byron Ayanoglu

Health

- 55 Most Common Medicinal Herbs Second Edition
  by Dr. Heather Boon, B.Sc.Phm., Ph.D. and Michael Smith, B.Pharm, M.R.Pharm.S., ND
- Canada's Baby Care Book
  by Dr. Jeremy Friedman MBChB, FRCP(C), FAAP, and Dr. Norman Saunders MD, FRCP(C)
- The Baby Care Book
  by Dr. Jeremy Friedman MBChB, FRCP(C), FAAP, and Dr. Norman Saunders MD, FRCP(C)
- Better Baby Food Second Edition
  by Daina Kalnins, MSc, RD, and Joanne Saab, RD
- Better Food for Pregnancy
  by Daina Kalnins, MSc, RD, and Joanne Saab, RD
- The Essential IBS Book
  by Dr. Alvin Newman, MD, FRCPC, FACP, FACG
- Crohn's & Colitis Diet Guide
  by Dr. A. Hillary Steinhart, MD, MSc, FRCP(C), and Julie Cepo, BSc, BASc, RD

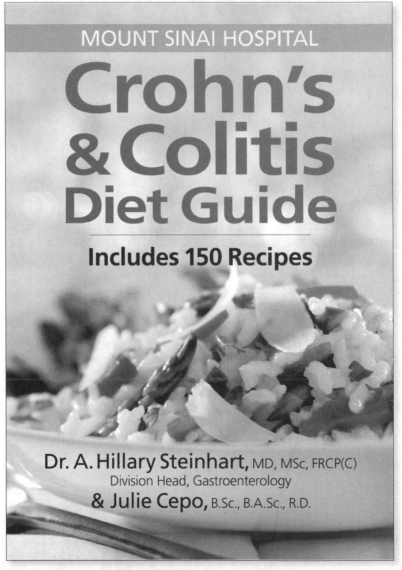